Sex, Edging and Orgasm: Delaying Orgasm for Better Sex

A Manual On Edging Techniques To Increase Arousal And Intensify Orgasms For Both Sexes

By

Patti W. Nieves

Sex, Edging and Orgasm 2

Copyright and Disclaimer:

© 2023 by Patti W. Nieves

consensual exploration while emphasizing the importance of communication, safety, and mutual consent in intimate relationships.

Every effort has been made to ensure the accuracy of the information presented. However, the author and publisher make no representations or warranties regarding the completeness, accuracy, or applicability of the contents. Readers are encouraged to verify information and seek professional advice when necessary.

By reading this book, the reader acknowledges and agrees to the terms outlined in this copyright and disclaimer notice.

About the Author - Patti W. Nieves

Patti W. Nieves is an accomplished content creator with a rich background in crafting insightful and engaging materials. With a keen understanding of the nuances of human connection and intimacy, Patti brings a unique perspective to the realm of sexual satisfaction.

As an experienced content creator, Patti has seamlessly blended her passion for writing with a genuine interest in the intricacies of relationships and pleasure. Through her work, she has contributed to the discourse on sexual well-being, providing valuable insights that resonate with readers seeking a deeper understanding of their desires.

Patti's commitment to fostering a positive and open dialogue surrounding sexual satisfaction is evident in her writings. Her work goes beyond conventional narratives, embracing a holistic approach that acknowledges the importance of emotional, psychological, and physical aspects of intimacy.

With a dedication to breaking down barriers and encouraging individuals to explore their own desires, Patti W. Nieves stands as a beacon in the field of sexual wellness content. Her writings serve as a source of empowerment, guiding readers toward a more fulfilling and satisfying journey of self-discovery and connection.

As an advocate for sexual satisfaction, Patti's work reflects not only her expertise as a content creator but also her genuine passion for helping individuals navigate the complexities of intimacy. Through her insightful contributions, she continues to inspire others to embrace a positive and open approach to their sexual well-being.

Table of content

Introduction

Meaning and Concept of Edging

The deliberate delaying or postponement of an orgasm during sexual arousal is referred to as "edging." It entails building to a climax and then purposefully decreasing or ceasing stimulation to maintain the elevated state of arousal. It is about engaging in sexual stimulation to the point of ejaculation before stopping and starting again. The idea behind this practice is that postponing an orgasm can result in more intense sexual experiences for partners as well as for the individual.

It will be essential to investigate the physiological and psychological effects of edging. The psychological aspect entails increasing the pleasure that comes from sexual activity and creating anticipation. Edging physiologically interacts with the body's arousal mechanism, permitting prolonged periods of increased sensitivity.

The Need to Push for Better Sexual Experience

Understanding the importance of edging establishes the framework for the entire manual. There are several advantages to edging, such as:

1. Enhanced Pleasure: People may have more intense orgasms and heightened sensations by extending their arousal, which can make for a more fulfilling sex.

2. Increased Intimacy: Edging promotes synchronization and communication between partners, which deepens their bond and helps them understand one another's desires.

3. Overcoming Challenges: Edging offers a useful strategy for addressing and overcoming these difficulties for people who struggle to achieve an orgasm or deal with premature ejaculation.

4. Mind-Body Connection: By introducing mindfulness into sexual encounters, Edging encourages people to be aware of and in the moment with their bodies, which enhances general wellbeing.

5. Variety in Sexual Expression: Individuals and couples can add variation to their sexual repertoire and maintain a dynamic and exciting intimacy by experimenting with different edging techniques.

By highlighting the significance of edging, the reader is encouraged to accept edging as a useful tool for improving their sex lives. This sets the stage for the ensuing discussion of techniques, obstacles, and advanced practices.

Chapter One: Understanding Arousal Processes

Physiological Aspects Arousal

A. Neurological Processes

Gaining knowledge of the neurological mechanisms underlying arousal can help one better understand the complex interactions between the brain and the nervous system during sex. The main neurological factors and how they affect the arousal process are shown below:

1. Arousal and Brain Regions:

Hypothalamus: The hypothalamus, which is frequently referred to as the brain's command center for sexual functions, is essential in initiating the release of sex hormones. It releases gonadotropin-releasing hormone (GnRH) in response to sexual stimuli, starting the hormonal chain reaction that leads to arousal.

Limbic System: The hippocampus and amygdala are two parts of this intricate network of brain structures that are essential for memory and emotional processing. The limbic system mediates emotional reactions to sexual stimuli, which affects the degree and caliber of arousal experiences. Pathways to Rewards: Reward-related brain circuitry, such as the nucleus accumbens, releases dopamine to reinforce positive experiences. These pathways are activated by sexual arousal, which results in a positive feedback loop that encourages people to seek out and partake in sexual activities.

2. Arousal and Neurotransmitters:

Dopamine: Dopamine, sometimes referred to as the "pleasure neurotransmitter," is released in reaction to sexual stimuli and plays a role in emotions of satisfaction and reward. Dopamine plays a crucial role in the neurological aspects of sexual response because elevated levels of the neurotransmitter during arousal enhance motivation and pleasure.

Serotonin: This neurotransmitter is involved in mood regulation and the inhibition of sexual response. Serotonin levels can change during arousal, which can affect the length and intensity of sexual experiences.

3. Genital Response and Neural Pathways:

Autonomic Nervous System (ANS): The involuntary body processes that are involved in sexual response are regulated by the ANS. Arousal causes the sympathetic nervous system to become active, which alters physiological processes including heart rate and blood flow to the genital area.

Pelvic Nerves: The pudendal and pelvic nerves, among other nerves, are involved in the transmission of signals from the genitalia to the brain. Knowing these neural pathways can help us understand how the brain interacts with the genitalia when we are aroused.

4. Hormonal Impact on Neurological Functions:

Estrogen and Testosterone: Sexual desire and response are influenced by sex hormones. While estrogen helps women's genital blood flow and lubrication, testosterone, which is found in both males and females, is linked to libido. These hormones fluctuate, which affects how the brain coordinates sexual arousal.

Through a thorough investigation of these brain functions, people can better comprehend the complex mechanisms regulating arousal. This information becomes especially important when discussing edging, since consciously tampering with these mechanisms permits a more complex and extended sensual experience.

B. Genital Response and Blood Flow

A fundamental viewpoint on the mechanics of sexual arousal can be gained by comprehending the physiological alterations in blood flow and genital response during arousal. Here we look at the complex physiological processes involved in sexual response, with a particular emphasis on the cardiovascular and genital domains.

A thorough grasp of the genital response and blood flow during arousal offers a comprehensive understanding of the physiological foundations of sexual experiences. For those who are interested in edging techniques, this information is fundamental because it enables a more deliberate and knowledgeable approach to extending and improving sexual pleasure.

1. Increased Blood Flow to Genital Areas:

Vasodilation, or the relaxation of blood vessels in response to sexual arousal, is an important physiological reaction. Increased blood flow to the genital areas—the penis in men and the clitoris and vaginal walls in women—is made possible by this process.

Erectile Tissue: An erection occurs when blood swells the spongy tissue of the penis in men. The body is primed for sexual activity by this increased blood flow, which also increases sensitivity.

Vaginal Lubrication: In females, the production of vaginal lubrication is stimulated by increased blood flow to the genital area. During sexual activity, this lubricant makes penetration more comfortable and lowers friction.

2. Role of Nitric Oxide

The signaling molecule in question Nitric Oxide (NO) is essential for vasodilation. NO is released in response to sexual stimuli, which encourages blood vessel smooth muscle cells to relax. Consequently, this improves blood flow to the genitalia.

Clitoral Erection and Penile Erection: In the case of the erectile response, NO is very important. By calming the smooth muscles in the erectile tissue, NO helps men achieve penile erection. Similarly, clitoral and vaginal engorgement in females are supported by increased NO production

3. Changes in the Cardiovascular System:

Increased Heart Rate: The sympathetic nervous system is activated by arousal, which raises heart rate. This increased heart rate makes sure that the body gets oxygen and nutrients in an effective manner, which supports the physiological processes related to sexual response.

Changes in Blood Pressure: There may be changes in blood pressure when one is sexually aroused. Even though modest increases are usual, people who have cardiovascular issues should be aware of these modifications and seek medical advice if needed.

4. The Significance of Blood Flow in Arousal and Edging:

Improving Sensitivity:The heightened sensitivity brought on by the increased blood flow to the genital areas amplifies the pleasurable sensations that accompany sexual activity. Edging helps people maintain this elevated sensitivity by extending arousal, which results in more fulfilling experiences.

Mastery and Control: For those who practice edging, knowing the dynamics of blood flow during arousal gives them more control over how they react. Through the manipulation of these physiological processes, people can improve their capacity to postpone the orgasm and extend the duration of the sexual encounter.

C. Hormonal Influence

Hormones are essential for controlling many aspects of sexual response, including arousal, desire, and general sexual function. Gaining knowledge of the hormonal dynamics during arousal can help one better appreciate the intricacy of the physiological mechanisms involved in sexual experiences. Hormonal influence is a complex facet of the physiological mechanisms linked to sexual arousal. When people integrate edging techniques into their intimate practices, they can better navigate and improve their sexual well-being because they have a thorough understanding of how hormones shape sexual experiences.

1. Testosterone: Although it is found in both sexes, testosterone is sometimes referred to as the "male hormone" because of its important role in enhancing libido and sexual desire. An increased inclination towards sexual activities is correlated with elevated testosterone levels.
Testosterone is necessary for men to maintain erectile function. Sufficient levels of testosterone promote the erectile tissue's reactivity to sexual stimuli, which helps erections occur and last.

2. Estrogen: One of the main female sex hormones, estrogen, helps to maintain genital blood flow. Sufficient levels of estrogen facilitate the genital region's blood vessels dilatation, which improves blood flow to the clitoris and vaginal walls. A key component of female sexual arousal, vaginal lubrication production is influenced by estrogen. During sexual activity, proper lubrication minimizes friction, improving comfort and pleasure.

3. Prolactin: After an orgasm, prolactin is released and linked to the refractory period, which is a period of time when people may become less responsive to sexual stimuli. For those who practice edging, knowing the function of prolactin is crucial

because it affects one's capacity to sustain arousal following an orgasm.

4. Oxytocin: Oxytocin, Often referred to as the "love hormone," is a hormone that is released during sexual activity and is linked to intimacy and bonding. Elevated oxytocin levels may improve the overall pleasure of sex as well as emotional connection.

5. Cortisol: The main stress hormone, cortisol, has an effect on sexual response. Arousal and libido may be affected by elevated cortisol levels, which are frequently linked to long-term stress. In order to preserve a healthy hormonal balance and encourage ideal sexual function, stress management is essential.

6. Hormonal Fluctuations: In females, hormonal changes during the menstrual cycle can affect sexual desire and responsiveness. Individuals and couples can navigate and embrace the natural ebb and flow of sexual interest by being aware of these variations.

7. Hormonal Influence on Edging: An understanding of hormonal dynamics helps edging practitioners maximize their levels of arousal.

People who know how hormones affect genital response, desire, and overall sexual function can adjust their edging techniques to coincide with changes in their hormones.

Psychological and Emotional Elements

A. Fantasy and Desire

Fantasy and desire are essential elements of the emotional and psychological terrain that mold the experience of sexual arousal. Gaining knowledge of these subtleties can help one better understand the intricate relationship between feelings and thoughts in relation to human sexuality.

Understanding and navigating these facets helps one gain a deeper comprehension of intimate relationship dynamics and one's own sexuality. A more complex and satisfying sexual journey may result from incorporating this awareness into the investigation of edging techniques.

1. Fantasy: Arousing scenarios or mental images are a part of sexual fantasies. These creative investigations can be more intricate and fantastical, or they can be mildly suggestive. Fantasies can heighten arousal and offer a creative outlet for sexual expression.

Fantasies vary greatly from person to person and are very individualized. They frequently represent the tastes, experiences, and aspirations of the individual. A nonjudgmental attitude toward one's own and other people's sexual imaginations is fostered by accepting the diversity of fantasies.

Because they stimulate the reward centers of the brain, fantasies have a big impact on arousal. Imaginary play can enhance pleasure and make a sexual encounter richer and more engaging.

2. Desire: One of the main internal drivers of intimate behavior is sexual desire. It includes a variety of emotions, ranging from a mild desire for intimacy to a strong need for physical contact. Understanding one's own sexuality requires investigating one's desires.

Desire is a dynamic concept that changes with time. The flow and ebb of desire are influenced by various factors, including relationship dynamics, stress, and mood. Understanding that desire is a flexible emotion enables people to adjust and express their needs to one another in a constructive way. Intimacy and an emotional bond between partners are fostered by open communication about desires.

A more fulfilling and satisfying sexual relationship is facilitated by mutual understanding and respect of each other's desires.

3. Relationship Between Fantasy and Desire: Fantasy and desire are related, with one frequently stoking the other. Vibrant fantasies can be sparked by strong desires, and fantasizing can both direct and intensify desires. The intricacy and richness of sexual experiences are enhanced by this interaction.

The efficacy of edging techniques can be increased by taking into account fantasies and understanding personal desires. During prolonged periods of arousal, fantasies can act as a mental stimulant, making the experience more fulfilling and prolonged.

4. Potential Challenges: Different fantasies or differing levels of desire may exist between partners. To resolve these differences, there needs to be open communication, empathy, and a readiness to consider mutual goals and limits.

Though fantasies can heighten arousal, it's crucial to strike a balance between reality and fantasy. The total satisfaction of sexual experiences may be impacted by unrealistic expectations derived from fantasies.

B. Mind-Body Relationships

An essential component of sexual experiences is the mind-body link, which affects how people experience, react to, and enjoy intimate moments. Understanding the complex interplay between the mind and body helps to understand how holistic sexual arousal and satisfaction are.

The mind-body connection is a dynamic and mutually reinforcing relationship that has a major impact on the psychological and emotional aspects of sexual experiences. Accepting this relationship can have a positive impact on one's general state of well-being and can be especially useful when learning and practicing edge techniques.

1. Conscious Awareness: Being fully present in the moment is a component of mindfulness, also known as conscious awareness. Mindfulness in the context of sexual experiences facilitates a deeper connection by enabling individuals to tune into sensations, emotions, and their partner's responses.

By minimizing distractions and anxieties, being mentally present during intimate moments allows people to fully participate in the sensory and emotional aspects of the experience. This increased attentiveness may lead to more gratifying and meaningful interactions.

2. Arousal and Emotional States: Sexual arousal is significantly influenced by emotions. Arousal can be aided or hindered by positive emotions like love and excitement as well as negative ones like stress and anxiety. Acknowledging and resolving emotional states enhances the quality of the sexual experience.
A partner's emotional connection to you enhances the whole sexual experience. Emotional connection creates a safe space for the exploration of fantasies and desires by fostering trust, vulnerability, and a sense of security.

3. Triggers for Psychological Arousal: Sexual arousal is strongly stimulated by the mind. Arousal can be elicited by ideas, memories, or mental images, demonstrating the complex relationship between mental operations and bodily reactions. Fantasy and desire-driven imagination is essential to psychological arousal. During sexual activities, using the imagination increases pleasure and makes the experience more dynamic and satisfying.

4. Mind-Body Techniques for Edging:.People often use mindful breathing as a mind-body technique when they edge. Throughout the process, taking deep, deliberate breaths can help control arousal levels, encourage relaxation, and improve general mindfulness. You can raise your level of arousal by focusing on particular feelings or by picturing desired situations. Edging practitioners frequently employ these methods to extend and enhance the pleasure that comes with having sex.

5. Cognitive Factors and Sexual Response: An individual's sexual response can be influenced by their personal views and beliefs about sex and their body. An improved mind-body connection leads to a more positive sexual experience; this is facilitated by positive attitudes and self-acceptance.
The thinking and behavior associated with sexuality are addressed by cognitive-behavioral methods. When dealing with issues like performance anxiety or low self-esteem, these strategies may help.

6. Post-Sexual Health: Beyond sexual activity, mind-body relationships also contribute to post-sexual health. Aftercare routines that involve emotional support and connection help to create a positive emotional fallout and improve the relationship between partners.

C. Social and Cultural Factors

Social and cultural factors have a significant impact on how people view, feel about, and express their sexuality. A thorough grasp of the complexities surrounding human intimacy can be obtained by looking at how cultural and societal factors affect the emotional and psychological aspects of sexual experiences.

Cultural and societal factors are ubiquitous factors that mold the emotional and psychological aspects of sexual experiences. To successfully navigate their own desires, promote healthy communication, and develop fulfilling intimate relationships within the framework of diverse cultural landscapes, individuals and couples must acknowledge and critically examine these influences.

1. Cultural Norms and Values: Social attitudes toward sexuality are determined by cultural norms, which have an impact on how people view and communicate their desires. The degree of openness and acceptance surrounding sexual topics can be influenced by varying cultural attitudes, which can range from conservative to liberal. People's roles and behaviors in sexual relationships are influenced by cultural expectations regarding gender roles.

Within intimate partnerships, these expectations can impact communication styles, power dynamics, and even the way in which desire is expressed.

2. Religious Views: Moral perspectives on sexuality are frequently shaped by religious teachings. Premarital sex, contraception, and other sexual practices can be viewed differently depending on cultural and societal adherence to religious beliefs.

Feelings of guilt or shame about sexual experiences that stray from accepted moral standards may be influenced by societal norms shaped by religious beliefs. People's general satisfaction and well-being may be impacted by this psychological effect.

3. Popular Culture and the Media: Images of sexuality in the media, such as television, movies, and advertisements, influence how society views sexuality. These representations have the power to mold expectations, sway desires, and reinforce ideals about body image, all of which can affect how people feel psychologically in close relationships.

The media's objectification of bodies and sexualization of people can affect how people see themselves, as well as how confident and at ease they are to express their sexuality. This in turn affects how emotionally healthy a person feels in sexual situations.

4. Awareness and Education: Programs for sexual education differ in terms of both content and quality among cultures and societies. Thorough sexual education promotes a healthier perspective on sexuality, lessens stigma, and helps people make informed decisions.
The degree to which people feel comfortable discussing their desires, boundaries, and preferences with partners is influenced by cultural norms surrounding communication about sex. Forging an emotional connection and navigating close relationships require open communication.

5. Cultural Diversity: Variations in sexual customs, rituals, and practices are accepted across cultural boundaries. Approaches to sexual diversity that are more accepting and inclusive are facilitated by an understanding of and respect for these distinctions. The way that people view their own sexual identity can be influenced by cultural and societal expectations. To promote self-acceptance and embrace a variety of sexual expressions, one must successfully navigate these influences.

6. Impact on Relationships: Power dynamics and communication styles in intimate relationships can be influenced by cultural and societal expectations. It takes awareness, communication, and respect for one another to navigate these dynamics. The expectations and dynamics of these relationships are affected by the prevalence of arranged marriages in some cultures. Emotional health depends on navigating and comprehending these cultural quirks.

D. Psychological Obstacles

Psychological obstacles can have a major impact on the psychological and emotional aspects of sexual experiences, posing difficulties that people may have to overcome. Promoting a fulfilling and healthy sexual life requires an understanding of these obstacles and solutions.

A satisfying and happy sexual experience depends on identifying and removing psychological barriers. Navigating and conquering these obstacles requires open communication, empathy, and a dedication to relationship and personal development.

1. Anxiety about Performance: Engaging fully in intimate moments can be impeded by anxiety related to one's sexual performance and fear of

being judged by a partner. This anxiety can have a detrimental effect on confidence and show up as self-doubt.

The pressure to live up to specific sexual expectations, whether internal or external, can exacerbate performance anxiety. Open communication, assurance, and an emphasis on enjoyment together rather than performance on an individual basis are frequently necessary to overcome these pressures.

2. Apprehensions Regarding Body Image: Those who battle with issues related to their bodies might feel inadequate or ashamed in private. It may be difficult to completely enjoy sexual experiences because of these worries. Being vulnerable with a partner or expressing desires can be made more difficult by having a negative body image. Overcoming this psychological barrier requires cultivating a positive body image and encouraging self-acceptance.

3. Previous Traumas: People who have endured past traumas, such as abuse or sexual assault, may be emotionally scarred, which impairs their capacity for intimacy and trust. Handling these situations calls for tact, encouragement, and frequent expert help. Psychological barriers to

arousal and pleasure during sexual encounters can result from traumatic experiences that cause flashbacks or triggers. Healing and overcoming these obstacles depend on establishing a secure and compassionate environment.

4. Fear of Rejection: Fear of exposing oneself emotionally to a partner can lead to fear of rejection. In close relationships, this fear may keep people from communicating their true selves or expressing their desires. Honest and transparent communication is essential to overcoming the fear of rejection. This psychological barrier is lessened by creating a supportive environment where partners feel comfortable communicating their needs and desires. This promotes emotional connection.

5. Religious and Cultural Guilt: Certain ideas or values may be ingrained in people through their cultural or religious upbringing, which can cause guilt or shame about one's sexual desires. Reconciling one's personal beliefs with one's own desires and values is necessary to overcome these obstacles. Self-worth and self-esteem can be severely impacted by cultural or religious guilt, which can psychologically prevent someone from embracing their sexuality. It could be important to

ask for help and have discussions that refute and challenge these beliefs.

6. Impaired Communication: A fulfilling sexual relationship may be hampered by difficulties in freely expressing boundaries and desires to a partner. Forging ahead through this obstacle, effective communication is a must. Differing sexual expectations between partners can cause annoyance and miscommunication.
Fostering a more positive emotional and psychological bond is facilitated by addressing these differences through candid communication and compromise.

7. Intimacy Fear: It can be difficult to build strong connections in intimate relationships if one is afraid of emotional intimacy and vulnerability. To break through this psychological barrier, one can gradually increase emotional intimacy and trust.

Openness to emotions may be difficult for people who have been betrayed or have had their trust violated in the past. To break through this barrier, it is imperative to restore trust and establish a safe environment.

A thorough understanding of arousal, including its physiological foundations as well as its emotional and psychological aspects, will enable readers to use edging techniques more skillfully. It emphasizes how the mind and body are connected during sexual experiences, setting the stage for the use of edging techniques in the manual's later sections.

Chapter Two: Edging Techniques For Men

Men's Step-by-Step Guide

A. Mindfulness and Relaxation:

People can enhance their experience and gain more control over their arousal levels by incorporating mindfulness and relaxation into each stage of the edging process. This all-encompassing strategy enhances one's overall sexual practices and cultivates a stronger mind-body connection.

Setting The Stage: First things first, pick an environment that encourages comfort and relaxation. Reduce the brightness, modify the interior temperature, and eliminate any possible disturbances. Set aside some time to mentally get ready for the edging session. Recognize any outside pressures and choose to put them aside for the duration of this time.

Important Mindfulness Ideas:
Adopt a non-judgmental mindset throughout the entire edge experience. Give up criticizing yourself and learn to accept the distinct feelings and reactions that come up.

Fix your attention on the here and now. Refrain from thinking about the past or projecting what will happen in the future. The edging experience is rich in the present. Throughout the practice, be kind and compassionate to yourself. Realize that every edging session is a chance for personal development and self-discovery.

B. Solo Exploration:
Understanding one's own responses and preferences through solo exploration is a crucial first step towards learning edging techniques. This section of the detailed instruction lays the groundwork for mastering arousal levels and improving the edging experience as a whole.

Alone exploration establishes the foundation for mastering the abilities and consciousness required for effective edging. Through mindfulness, openness, and self-discovery, people can lay a strong foundation for advanced edging techniques and increased sexual well-being during this phase of life.

Ideas For Solo Exploration
Curiosity and Openness: Have an inquisitive and receptive mindset when embarking on solo exploration. Without any expectations or

preconceptions, give yourself permission to investigate your body's reactions.

Non-Judgmental Observation: When solo edging, practice non-judgmental observation of your thoughts, feelings, and sensations. This kind of thinking makes it easier to accept who you are, which makes the experience more fulfilling and happy.

Privacy and Comfort: When exploring alone, pick a space that is both quiet and cozy. Assure yourself that you won't be disturbed, establishing a secure environment for introspection. To establish an environment that encourages rest and concentrated exploration, take into account elements like lighting, temperature, and ambience.

When incorporating sexual fantasies into your solo exploration, do so with awareness. Pay attention to the feelings and images that the fantasies bring to mind. Recognize the impact they have on arousal levels. Spend some time thinking back on the solo exploration session. Think about the methods or strategies that worked best, and note any new information you discovered while exploring.

Exploration:Self-Compassion: Treat yourself with kindness and compassion while you're exploring. Accept and love yourself as you are as you embark on your self-discovery path.

Progress and Patience: Recognize that becoming an expert at edging techniques takes time. Enjoy your accomplishments and practice self-compassion while you continue to hone your ability.

Flexibility: Remain open to modifying your strategy in light of changing responses and preferences. Accept the fact that solo exploration is dynamic and modify your methods accordingly.

C. Stimulation Build-Up:

By progressively raising arousal, gaining control, and producing a more complex and customized experience, stimulation build-up is the cornerstone of effective edging. With deliberate pacing and careful investigation, people gradually build stimulation.

1. Sensory Awareness: Start the session with a mildly stimulating environment. This could entail gentle touches that gradually raise arousal, such as strokes or light caresses. Concentrate on being totally present and aware of your body's sensations.

Observe the body's reaction to touch and the minute changes in arousal that occur when stimulation is applied.

2. Gradual Intensity: Gradually raise the level of stimulation as the session goes on. This may entail experimenting with various pressure, speed, or focused touch settings. Observe how arousal changes in response to greater stimulation. The next steps of the edging practice should be guided by your awareness of any areas that are more sensitive or pleasurable.

3. Exploration of the Erogenous Zone: Examine the body's various erogenous zones. These can include parts that react well to touch, such as the inner thighs, neck, chest, and other areas. Track the responses of various erogenous zones to stimulation. Acknowledge that every individual might possess distinct regions of elevated sensitivity, and this exploration adds to a more customized edging encounter.

4. Incorporating Mental Focus: Increase the level of stimulation by adding mental focus as arousal increases. This could entail visualizing fantasies or desires or practicing mindful awareness of the sensations that are happening right now.

Reflect and consider the stimulation modalities that were most enjoyable or successful after the session. Future edging procedures should take these preferences into account. Be willing to modify your stimulation methods in response to changing preferences. The exploration and adaptation process adds to a more fulfilling and customized edging experience.

Important Points to Remember
Communication with Partner: Be honest about preferences and feelings when practicing edging with a partner. This kind of cooperation builds mutual understanding and improves the experience as a whole.

Regular Practice: The ability to build up stimulation is one that gets better with regular practice. Frequent edging sessions help with the gradual development of control and increased pleasure.

Patience and Exploration: Approach the building of stimulation with a spirit of exploration and patience. Accept the process of self-discovery and acknowledge that as you continue to hone your edging skills, your preferences may change.

D. Controlled Pacing:

One of the most important skills in learning edging techniques is controlled pacing, which enables people to deliberately move between arousal levels. People can hone this ability and improve their overall edging practice by combining reflective adaptation, breath synchronization, and rhythmic pacing.

1. Creating a Rhythm: Once arousal starts, create a rhythm that suits your comfort zone. Start the pacing mindfully, considering your body's reaction and the level of stimulation. Pacing should be started deliberately; avoid making quick or hurried movements. This establishes the framework for a deliberate and controlled edging session.

2. Regular and Steady Build-Up: Continue to gradually and steadily increase stimulation. By gradually increasing arousal, this methodical approach keeps you aware of your body's reactions. Observe carefully how your body reacts to the pace. To keep things under control, take note of any areas where you feel more sensitive and modify the rhythm accordingly.

3. Breath Synchronization: Match the pace of your breathing. Breathe in a rhythmic pattern that

balances the level of stimulation. Harmonious mind-body connection is enhanced by this synchronization. During the pacing, stay conscious of your breathing. This mindful breathing reduces stress and acts as a tool to control arousal.

4. Tracking Orgasmic Proximity: Regularly assess your level of arousal. Recognize how close you are to experiencing an orgasm. Pacing changes can be made on time thanks to this constant observation. Develop the ability to spot early indicators of an impending orgasm. This ability becomes essential for putting deliberate stops or intensity reductions into practice when necessary.

5. Intentional Pauses or Reductions: Incorporate purposeful pauses or intensity reductions as you get close to an orgasm. This calculated pause breaks the flow and keeps the action from building quickly to a climax. Savor the silence that occurs during the break. Before picking up the pace again, give your body some time to calm down and utilize this to regain control over your arousal levels.

6. Gradual Resumption: After the deliberate pause, gradually pick up the pace again. Re-enter the rhythm while paying closer attention to how your body reacts. When modifying the pacing, take into

account the input from the deliberate pause. The key to improving control over arousal is to repeat this iterative process of pacing, pausing, and starting again.

7. Iterative Learning: Consider how well the pacing strategy worked after each session. Decide what went well and what needs to be improved. Iterative learning is aided by this reflective process. Be willing to change your pacing to accommodate changing needs and reactions. The secret to mastering controlled pacing in edging is the ability to modify and improve your approach.

8. Incorporate Mental Focus: During the session, incorporate mental focus as you go at your own pace. This may be as simple as visualizing what you want or practicing mindful awareness of your current feelings. Make sure that the integration of mental and physical engagement is balanced. The pace of the mind and body should be in harmony. In order to improve the overall depth and satisfaction of the edging experience, try to create a harmonious connection between the two.

9. Maintain Consistency in Pacing Throughout Cycles: Follow a methodical and constant pace during the edging cycles. A session's flow should

not be disturbed by sudden changes in intensity. Take pace as a skill that can be developed through regular practice. Your ability to manage the fine line between arousal and control will improve with practice in controlled pacing.

10. Communication with a Partner: When practicing edging with a partner, keep lines of communication open regarding the pace. Talk about likes, criticism, and any changes that should be made to improve the experience for everyone. Work together with your partner to adjust the pacing according to your mutual comfort and preferences. A mutual comprehension enhances the synchronization and enjoyment of the edging exercise.

Important Guidelines for Controlled Pacing: Conscious Presence: Adopt a mindful presence while maintaining a controlled pace. Pay close attention to the present, pay attention to your body's reactions, and pay attention to the session's rhythm.

Patience and perseverance are required because mastering controlled pacing takes time. Recognize that it will take time and consistent effort to hone this skill, so practice patience and persistence.

Adaptability and Exploration: Approach things with flexibility and be willing to learn new things. Try out various pacing techniques to see which one suits you the best and makes for a satisfying edging experience.

E. Breath Control:
Breath control is a fundamental component of the methodical instruction manual for men who practice edging. Through the practice of awareness-building, pacing synchronization, and arousal adaptation, people can use their breath to increase their control and enjoyment during the edging session.

1. Conscious Initiation: Focus on your breathing at the start of the edging session. Before you intentionally begin practicing controlled breathing, take a few moments to observe your natural breathing pattern. Give your body time to adjust to the deliberate rhythm of controlled breathing by making the shift gradually.

2. Synchronization with Pacing: Align the pace of stimulation with your breathing. Regardless of how fast or slow the beat is going, make sure your breath is in sync with the beat to create a synchronized experience. Breathe differently as the level of

stimulation varies. If your breathing quickens, then take more breaths; if it slows down, then let your breathing also slow down.

3. Rhythmic Breathing: Establish a breathing pattern that synchronizes with the edging session's tempo and intensity. Throughout the process of raising arousal, this steady rhythm acts as a stabilizing anchor. Aim for regularity in your breathing pattern. Throughout the session, the mindful approach helps to maintain a sense of stability and control.

4. Breath Awareness: Throughout the entire session, stay mindful of your breath at all times. By considering the inhalation and exhalation as essential elements of the whole experience, you can cultivate a sense of presence. To connect the mental and physical facets of the edging exercise, use your breath. Being mindful of your breathing strengthens the link between your mind and body and creates a more engaging experience.

5. Depth of Breaths: Try different breathing depths. Think about taking deeper breaths to help you relax and avoid tension during times when your arousal is high. Depending on how aroused you are, adjust the depth of your breaths. During times of high

stimulation, shallow breathing can help with increased sensitivity and control.

6. Breath Pause During Intentional Breaks: Take a brief breath pause during the introduction of intentional breaks in the edging session. Let your breath come in and out, establishing a little moment of calm and equilibrium. During breaks, the breath pause helps you regain your composure. It keeps things from quickly spiraling out of control and adds to the deliberate, regulated aspect of the whole edging experience.

7. Gradual Breath Adjustments: Pay attention to changes in your arousal levels during the session and gradually modify your breathing. This flexibility helps to keep arousal under control. Breathe continuously, adjusting its depth and pace in response to the changing dynamics of the edging cycles.

8. Post-Session Reflection: Consider the function of breath control following the edging session. Think about how your breathing affected the whole experience and note any observations or insights about how it affected your level of control and arousal. To incorporate better breath control into upcoming edging sessions, use reflections. Think

about how modifying your breathing techniques
can lead to a more streamlined and fulfilling
routine.

Important Guidelines for Breath Control:
Mindful Presence: Approaching breath control
mindfully is important. Give your full attention to
the rhythm of your breathing, and make use of it as
a tool to improve control and awareness.
Adaptability: Let your breath be as flexible as you
are. As a result, it will adapt to variations in tempo,
intensity, and arousal levels, encouraging a
dynamic and adaptable practice.

Integration with Other Techniques: Acknowledge
that breath control is a crucial component of the
edging process as a whole. For a comprehensive
approach, smoothly incorporate it with other
strategies like pacing, deliberate breaks, and mental
engagement.

F. Introduce Fantasy:
Adding fantasy to the edging experience enhances
the overall journey of pleasure and self-discovery by
adding a layer of complexity and depth.
People can use fantasy to increase arousal and
make edging more fulfilling if they approach it

mindfully, adaptably, and with an emphasis on personalization.

1.Gradually Integration: Consciously introduce fantasy as arousal increases. This may be imagining situations, pulling memories from memory, or creating mental images consistent with what you want. Gradually incorporate fantasy so that it becomes a part of the whole experience. A smooth transition between the physical experiences of the edging session and mental engagement is guaranteed by this mindful start.

2. Alignment with Arousal Levels: Throughout the edging cycle, match the arousal levels with the fantasy's introduction. To maximize the overall intensity and pleasure, introduce it when arousal is at its highest. Be flexible with the introduction of fantasy based on personal tastes. While some people find it more effective to engage during the peak of arousal, others might prefer to engage early.

3. Rich sensory and visual details should be incorporated into the fantasy. Activate the mind with vivid imagery that heightens arousal and improves the overall sensory experience. To explore your fantasies and desires, use fantasy as a tool. Let

the mind wander, exploring individual inclinations that lead to increased enjoyment.

4. Maintaining Balance with Physical Sensations: While immersed in fantasy, stay mindful of the physical sensations experienced during the edging session. Steer clear of total dissociation and make sure the mental activity complements the tactile experience rather than takes its place. Aim for a harmonious ratio of the mental to the physical. The combination of fantasy and physical sensations makes for a more fulfilling and engaging edging experience.

5. Gradual Escalation with Fantasy: As the edging session goes on, gradually increase the fantasy's level of intensity. Make use of fantasy as a tool to increase arousal, investigate various scenarios, and enhance enjoyment in general. Based on your body's feedback, dynamically adjust the fantasy's intensity. This flexibility makes sure that fantasy doesn't become a hindrance but rather a helpful component.

6. Sensual Words and Images: Incorporate sensual words and images into your fantasy. Describe situations or conjure up images that appeal to several senses, enhancing the immersive quality of

the mental experience. To increase arousal, mentally or vocally narrate the fantasy. Using descriptive language makes the experience in the mind more vivid and engaging.

Important Guidelines for Introducing Fantasy: Customization: Adapt the dream to your own tastes and aspirations. The mental engagement becomes more authentic and effective because of this personalization.

Open Exploration: Have an exploratory and open mind when approaching fantasy. Give yourself permission to explore a range of situations and topics, accepting the multiplicity of aspirations that enhance a satisfying edging experience.

Maintain a strong mind-body connection when introducing fantasy. For an edging practice to be holistic and fulfilling, mental engagement and physical sensations must work in harmony.

Exploring Different Approaches to Delay Orgasm

A. Start-Stop Technique:

By exploring between sexual stimulation and deliberate pauses, the Start-Stop Technique helps delay orgasms. This technique actively manages and prolongs the duration of sexual pleasure, this technique empowers people and promotes heightened awareness of arousal levels.

1. Start of Stimulation: Start with a sexually stimulating activity, such as self-stimulation or partner stimulation. As you progressively increase intensity, maintain a regular rhythm of arousal.

2. Timely Pause: Intentionally turn off stimulation just before an impending orgasm reaches the point of no return. During this little respite, let the arousal decrease.

3. Resume Stimulation: Continue the cycle of sexual stimulation following the pause. The secret is to build control over climax by navigating the edge of arousal.

4. Repetition and Mastery: Throughout a session, repeat the start-stop cycles. People can become

more in control over time, which improves their capacity to postpone orgasm.

B. Apply Squeeze Method:
The Squeeze Technique involves stopping sexual stimulation in order to postpone orgasm.
By interfering just before an orgasm, this technique offers a useful way for people or partners to actively control and prolong the duration of sexual activity.

1. Initiation of Stimulation: Start a sexually stimulating relationship, either with a partner or on your own. Pay special attention to the feelings as arousal increases.

2. Determine the Point of No Return: Find the moment just prior to the verge of an orgasm. To identify this threshold, awareness is essential.

3. Squeeze Action: Stop stimulation after determining the point of no return.
Press firmly on the base of the penis for approximately 30 seconds using your thumb and forefinger.

4. Release and Resume: Let go of the tension and give the arousal some time to fade. Get back into the sexual game, repeating the steps as necessary.

5. Enhanced Control Over Time: Consistent application of the squeeze technique can result in increased ejaculation control. The squeeze can be applied jointly by partners, forming a shared strategy.

C. Pelvic Floor Exercises:

Exercises for the pelvic floor, also referred to as Kegel exercises, can be used to postpone orgasm. Exercises targeting the pelvic floor provide a non-invasive, natural way for people to actively work and strengthen the muscles that control ejaculation, which can prolong the duration of sexual pleasure.

1. Identifying Pelvic Floor Muscles: To start, note which muscles in the pelvic floor are in charge of ejaculation. Try to halt the urine's flow midstream to identify these muscles.

2. Isometric Contractions: Work on your pelvic floor muscles through isometric contractions. Squeeze, then hold for a short while before releasing these muscles.

3. Regular Exercise Schedule: Create a pelvic floor exercise schedule that is consistent. Over time, progressively lengthen the contractions.

4. Incorporate During Arousal: Incorporate pelvic floor
exercises during intercourse. To postpone
ejaculation as an orgasm approaches, tense your
pelvic floor muscles.

5. Enhanced Control: Regular exercise helps
improve pelvic floor muscle control. This increased
control helps to prolong sexual activity by delaying
ejaculation.

D. Pay Attention to Other Feelings:

One way to delay an orgasm is to focus on other
sensations. Diverting attention by concentrating on
other feelings enables people to postpone an
orgasm by expanding their awareness beyond
genital stimulation.

1. Mindful Distraction: As an orgasm approaches,
shift focus away from genital sensations. Pay
attention to other body parts or the sensory
experience as a whole.

2. Take A Look at Non-Genital Stimulation
Try stimulating your body in ways other than the
genitalia, like petting other areas.
Activities that increase arousal in general but do not
directly target the genitalia should be undertaken.

3. Cognitive Diversion: Pass your time contemplating non-sexual subjects by using cognitive diversion. The time to climax can be extended by shifting one's mental focus.

4. Differentiating Stimuli: Introduce novel experiences, such as temperature variations or textures. An orgasm may be delayed by a variety of stimuli.

Develop a robust mind-body connection when engaging in sexual activities. Individuals can expand the total experience by being aware of and present for a variety of sensations.

E. Patterns of Masturbation:
Delaying orgasm can be achieved by altering one's masturbation patterns.
Individuals can delay orgasm during solo sexual activities by intentionally altering their technique, pacing, and mental engagement during masturbation. This process is known as adaptation of masturbation patterns.

1. Differing Stimulation Methods: Try out various hand motions, pressures, and strokes when self-stimulation.

Changing patterns can help avert predictability and postpone the big moment.

2. Controlled Pacing: Pace consciously when you're masturbating. Slowly increase arousal, halt, and then resume in a manner similar to the start-stop method.

3. Incorporate Edging: Practice edging during solo sessions. Bring yourself close to orgasm, pause, and then repeat, building control over climax.

4. Mindful Breath Integration: Coordinate deliberate breathing with patterns of masturbation. Controlling arousal and delaying an orgasm can be achieved with mindful breathing.

5. Erogenous Zone Exploration: During self-stimulation, consider exploring additional erogenous zones. By dividing attention, this variety may help postpone orgasm.

6. Fantasy Integration: Incorporate fantasies and mental activity while masturbating. This gives the experience a cognitive component that may postpone the climax.

Tips for Enhancing Pleasure While Edging

1. High-quality Lubricant: To improve feelings, pick a lubricant of superior quality. This makes the experience more enjoyable overall in addition to reducing friction.

2. Temperature Play: Try edging while experimenting with temperature changes, such as warm or cool feelings. This may add another level of perceptual stimulation.

3. Incorporate Sex Toys: Add sex toys to the procedure of edging. Other gadgets, like vibrators, can heighten enjoyment and offer extra stimulation.

4. Partner Communication: When experimenting with a partner, keep lines of communication open regarding preferences, boundaries, and desires. This mutual comprehension makes the whole experience better.

5. Erotic Literature or Media: Include erotic literature or media in your daily edging routine. This can pique mental interest and make the experience more enjoyable and immersive.

6. Try Various Positions: Changing up your sexual posture can offer a variety of experiences and enhance your edging experience. Finding positions that postpone climax increases practice diversity.

7. Sensual Touch: During the edging procedure, use tender touches and caresses. This enhances the overall experience by providing both sensual and emotional fulfillment.

8. Discover Tantric Practices: Get knowledge about tantric techniques that are aimed at extending pleasure. Extended arousal can be facilitated by methods like energy circulation and regulated breathing.

9. Relaxation and Hydration: Make sure to get enough rest and maintain a healthy weight. A more pleasurable edging experience is correlated with maintaining general well-being.

10. Celebrate Progress: Celebrate the advancements made in edging techniques. Any improvement in self-control and extended enjoyment is a worthy accomplishment.

For men, edging can be more rewarding and satisfying when they follow these step-by-step instructions, experiment with different orgasm-delaying techniques, and incorporate pleasure-enhancing tips. Recall that developing your edging skills over time requires both patience and self-discovery.

Chapter Three: Edging Techniques For Women

Women-Specific Edging Practices

A. Clitoral Edging:

This method of clitoral stimulation emphasizes control, variation, and synchronization with breath and pacing to produce heightened satisfaction and prolonged pleasure. It is a deliberate and mindful approach.

1. Controlled Stimulation: By using varied and controlled clitoral stimulation, arousal can be gradually built. Try out various patterns, pressures, and speeds.

2. Pacing and Rhythm: Create a stimulating rhythm that matches your level of comfort and arousal. Strive for deliberate pacing, building to a climax before letting up.

3. Sensory Exploration: Take in the clitoral hood and its environs as well as the whole area. Change up the feelings you experience to find what increases arousal without pushing for an orgasm.

4. Incorporate mindful breathing into clitoral stimulation. Use deliberate breathing to control arousal and encourage calm.

5. Intentional Pauses: Before the orgasmic point, introduce deliberate pauses in the clitoral stimulation process. Permit excitement to fade for a little while before continuing, prolonging enjoyment.

6. Practice Mindful Awareness: Throughout clitoral edging, remain alert and mindful of your feelings. The mind-body connection is strengthened by mindfulness, which makes life more satisfying.

B. Exploration of Erogenous Zones:
In women-specific edging practices, erogenous zone exploration entails a thorough approach to sensual stimulation and touch, encouraging a more satisfying and expansive journey towards prolonged pleasure.

1. All-Inclusive Sensual Exploration: Venture past the clitoris and discover diverse erogenous zones throughout the body. Try soft caresses, kisses, or touches to find out which parts of your body are more aroused.

2. Nipple Stimulation: The nipples are a noticeable area of erogenous stimulation. To improve overall pleasure, adjust the nipple stimulation's pattern and intensity.

3. Inner Thigh Sensation: Try kissing and softly touching your inner thighs. Build up to the genital area gradually to create anticipation.

4. Neck and Ear Stimulation: Check for increased sensitivity in the neck and ears. Arousal can be increased by soft breath, nibbles, or gentle kisses.

5. Lower Abdomen and Pelvic Area: Give the lower abdomen and pelvic area some gentle pressure. These kinds of sensations can enhance clitoral stimulation for a more comprehensive experience.

6. Full-Body Connection: When engaging in sensual exploration, try to establish a full-body connection. Connecting different erogenous zones results in an edging experience that is longer and more immersive.

C. Internal Stimulation Techniques:

In women-specific edging practices, internal stimulation techniques entail a deliberate and varied approach to investigating vaginal sensations, promoting prolonged pleasure and a more profound sense of connection with one's own body.

1. Try Out Different Finger Techniques: Explore various finger motions for inner stimulation. Experiment with depth, pressure, and speed to see what makes the most sense.

2. Introduce Sex Toys: Include toys meant to stimulate the internal climax. For more pleasure, try varying the sizes, shapes, and vibration patterns.

3. Pay Attention to the G-Spot: The vagina's anterior wall is home to the G-spot. Try focusing stimulation to increase arousal and extend enjoyment.

4. Upward and Circular Motions: When you experience internal stimulation, move upward or in circles. These motions have the potential to elicit a wide range of feelings and prolong arousal.

5. Integrate External and Internal Stimulation:
Incorporate both external and internal erogenous
zones into your stimulation simultaneously. This
combination promotes prolonged arousal and
increases overall pleasure.

6. Mindful Exploration: Use awareness and
mindfulness when addressing internal stimulation.
Pay attention to your body's reactions and modify
your methods according to personal taste.

D. Mindful Breathing and Relaxation:

For a more prolonged and fulfilling experience,
women-specific edging practices that incorporate
mindful breathing and relaxation techniques offer a
comprehensive approach that fosters a calm mental
state and heightened awareness of bodily
sensations.

1. Conscious Breath Initiation: Concentrate on
conscious, purposeful breathing to start the edging
session. To induce calm, take a deep breath, letting
it fill your lungs, and then slowly exhale.

2. Synchronized Breathing with Stimulation:
Coordinate your breathing with your sexual or
sensual cues. To create a harmonious connection,

time your inhalations and exhalations to the
rhythm of touch or arousal.

3. Breath as a Sensory Anchor: When edging, use
your breath as a sensory anchor. To stay calm and
in control even when feelings become more intense,
bring your attention back to your breathing.

4. Gradual Breath Adjustments: Depending on your
level of arousal, gradually change the depth and
pace of your breathing. When arousal is high,
taking deep breaths can help you relax and avoid
getting tense.

5. Mindful Pause with Breath: Use the moment to
engage in a quick mindful pause while introducing
deliberate pauses in stimulation. During these
times, pay attention to your breathing and give your
body time to calm down before continuing.

6. Exhalation for Release: Give special attention to
the breath's exhalation phase to create a feeling of
release. When edging, this technique can help you
stay mentally and physically at ease.

7. Gradual-Relaxation Methods: During the edging
session, incorporate progressive relaxation
techniques. Reduce overall tension by

concentrating on methodically relaxing various muscle groups.

8. Incorporate Optimal Thoughts into Every Breath Cycle: Include uplifting statements into every breath cycle. For an even better edging experience, use affirmations that are linked to relaxation, pleasure, and self-acceptance.

Incorporating Edging into Solo and Coupled Experiences

A. Solo Edging:

This practice gives people the chance to get in close contact with their own desires, investigate arousal reactions, and hone strategies that lead to sustained pleasure.

1. Personalized Exploration: When solo edging, one explores their own body and arousal levels on a personal level. Based on your own preferences, try out different methods, speeds, and stimulation levels.

2. Creating a Cozy Space: Establish a cozy, personal space for lone edging. Make sure there is room for unwinding, concentration, and leisurely exploration.

3. Mindful Self-Awareness: When solo edging, cultivate mindful self-awareness. Develop a closer relationship with yourself by being aware of your breath, sensations, and arousal levels.

4. Integration of Techniques: Combine several edging methods, such as internal stimulation, erogenous zone exploration, and clitoral stimulation. Combine methods to find a customized and satisfying edging regimen.

5. Fantasy Experimentation: Individual fantasies can be explored through solo edging. Increase arousal and prolong pleasure by introducing mental engagement, visualization, or fantasies.

6. Managed Pacing and Intervals: Engage in deliberate pacing by building tension to a near-climax and then reducing it. Include pauses to slow down the rate of escalation and lengthen the edging session.

7. Mindful Breath Integration: Coordinate mindful breathing with edging exercises. To control your arousal levels and maintain present-moment awareness, use your breath as a tool.

B. Partnered Edging:
This activity takes couples on a personal journey of discovery, enjoyment, and bonding. Both partners can have a satisfying experience when there is open communication and a willingness to try new things.

1. Open Communication: Discuss edging preferences, boundaries, and desires in an open and honest manner with your partner. An atmosphere of mutual understanding fosters partnered edging.

2. Shared Exploration: Examine each other's bodies and reactions together. Try varying methods, timing, and degrees of stimulation to find out what makes you more happy.

3. Mutual Edging Practices: To promote a reciprocal experience, take turns edging one another. A mutual understanding of pacing and pleasure is developed through this reciprocal engagement.

4. Feedback and Adjustments: During partnered edging, give and receive feedback. Make necessary adjustments to techniques based on nonverbal and verbal cues to guarantee that both partners are happy.

5. Breath Synchronization: When you're edging, match your partner's breathing patterns. A more immersive experience is facilitated by coordinated breathing, which also strengthens intimacy and connection.

6. Incorporating Fantasy: During partnered edging, introduce shared fantasies or engage in mutual mental engagement. This gives the experience a cognitive component that makes it more enjoyable for both partners.

7. Combination of Techniques: Mix and match different edging methods, such as internal stimulation, erogenous zone exploration, and clitoral stimulation. Combining different techniques makes both partners feel more satisfied overall.

8. Respect for Boundaries: Make sure that everyone is aware of and respectful of one another's limits. A good partnered edging experience requires a secure and consenting environment.

C. Mutual Edging Exploration:

By encouraging shared enjoyment, communication, and a greater comprehension of one another's desires, mutual edging exploration fortifies the bond between partners.

1. Shared Responsibilities: Mutual edging calls for shared accountability for the enjoyment of each partner. The edging experience involves active participation from both partners.

2. Taking Turns: To promote reciprocity, partners edge one another in turn. Mutual understanding of pacing, preferences, and arousal is improved by this practice.

3. Establish Clear Channels for Verbal and Nonverbal Communication: Make sure that all communication is clear. To assist each other in guiding their edging techniques, partners offer suggestions and remarks.

4. Harmonization of Beats: During mutual edging, harmonize your bodily and respiratory rhythms. Breath and well-coordinated motions strengthen the bond.

5. Joint Technique Exploration: Examine several edging methods in tandem. Together, explore the erogenous zone, play with clitoral stimulation, and engage in internal stimulation.

6. Collaborative Fantasy Exploration: Take part in mutual edging or exchange fantasies. In order to enhance the experience and strengthen the bond, mutual fantasy exploration is added.

7. Respect for Partner's Boundaries: Give each other's comfort zones and boundaries top priority. For mutual edging exploration to be constructive and enjoyable, a consensual environment is essential.

D. Community and Feedback:
In order to improve and refine edging experiences, the community's involvement and feedback are essential. A collaborative and encouraging approach makes the process of edging more rewarding, whether it is done alone, with a partner, or by looking for advice online.

1. Online Communities and Resources: Look for websites or online groups devoted to edging techniques. Sites that promote conversation, guidance, and experience sharing can offer insightful information.

2. Gaining Knowledge from Others: Talk to people who have dealt with edging before. Gaining insights, methods, and viewpoints for solo and

partnered edging can be obtained by studying the experiences of others.

3. Giving and Receiving Feedback: Foster an environment where both individual and group edging experiences value feedback. To make future sessions better, let's hear about your preferences, areas for improvement, and best practices.

4. Collaborative Exploration: If you have a partner who is willing to experiment and communicate, think about exploring edging techniques together. Coupled feedback makes the experience more personalized and fulfilling for both parties.

5. Encourage an Open Discussion about Desires, Boundaries, and Preferences: Create a Supportive Environment. Edging can be comfortably explored by individuals and partners in a nonjudgmental space.

6. Thinking Back on Experiences: Consider your own and other people's edging experiences. Think about the things that were easy, hard, or that could be changed for next sessions.

7. Constant Improvement: Adopt an attitude where edging techniques are always being improved. Individual or partner feedback is an invaluable resource for improving methods and increasing satisfaction.

8. Sharing Insights and Resources: Provide partners or the community with insights and resources. Adding to a group's body of knowledge encourages cooperation and mutual development in edging techniques.

Overcoming Challenges for Women in Edging

A. Address Mental Blocks

In order to address mental blocks in women's edging experiences, a comprehensive strategy that includes self-awareness, communication, cultivating a positive mindset, cultural analysis, education, and, when required, professional support must be used. Establishing a setting that promotes self-acceptance, empowerment, and a healthy relationship with one's own sexuality is the aim.

1. Awareness and Acceptance: Realize that mental obstacles resulting from cultural norms, individual

inhibitions, or prior experiences can affect women just as much as they do everyone else. Recognize that these difficulties are common and manageable. Recognize that each woman's experience with edging is distinct. Accept the range of needs and experiences, and grant each person's preference without passing judgment.

2. Communication and Self-Expression: Encourage honest dialogue about expectations, boundaries, and desires with both yourself and, if relevant, your partner. Creating a secure environment for communication aids in overcoming mental obstacles. Promote introspection and self-expression. Without social constraints restricting their autonomy, women ought to feel free to express their needs and take an interest in their bodies.

3.Healthy Body Image and Mindset: Advocate for self-love and body positivity. Promote body positivity by acknowledging that a range of body types and appearances are attractive and natural. Dispel cultural myths and conventions that could lead to a poor perception of one's body. Develop an attitude that honors self-acceptance and recognizes each woman's individuality.

4. Cultural Norms and Influences: Recognize the cultural influences that could lead to mental blockages. Identify and question cultural norms that have the potential to affect how women view their sexuality and desires.
Pursue empowerment by being cognizant of culture. Accept cultural elements that uphold and honor women's independence, encouraging a healthy relationship with one's sexuality.

5. Education and Exploration: Get informational materials about women's pleasure and sexual health. Women who possess knowledge are better able to combat false information and debunk myths that cause mental obstacles. Promote introspection and self-learning. A more positive and knowledgeable approach to edging can be achieved by breaking down mental barriers and having a better understanding of one's own anatomy, desires, and responses.

6. Advise and Assistance: If mental obstacles don't go away, think about getting help from a therapist or counselor. Mental health specialists can offer customized approaches to tackle particular issues and encourage a positive outlook. Develop understanding and supportive relationships when participating in partnered experiences. Partners are

essential in fostering an atmosphere that values candid dialogue and reciprocal inquiry.

7. Advantageous Feedback: No matter how small the progress, acknowledge it and celebrate it. Positive reinforcement can help people see themselves more favorably and gain confidence in their capacity to get past mental obstacles. Promote introspection on one's own development and accomplishments. Women can keep journals of their experiences, recording their victories over mental health issues and moments of empowerment.

B. Understanding Women's Unique Physiology: Overcoming obstacles associated with edging requires a fundamental understanding of women's unique physiology. Women can create a positive and fulfilling experience that is in line with their unique physiological characteristics by integrating knowledge, self-exploration, adaptability to hormonal fluctuations, and open communication.

1. Female Anatomy Knowledge: Gain a thorough understanding of the clitoris, labia, vagina, and pelvic floor muscles as well as other aspects of female anatomy first. Gaining knowledge enables

women to establish a physiological connection with their bodies.
Promote self-discovery to become acquainted with one's own anatomy. This practical experience makes for a more customized and knowledgeable edging strategy.

2. Physiological Variability: Recognize that women differ physiologically from one another. Since every body reacts to stimulation differently, what works for one individual might not work for another. Stress the value of learning about individual preferences. Because every woman's physiological reactions are unique, edging techniques must be customized for each individual.

3. Awareness of Cycles: Recognize the effects of changing hormone levels during the menstrual cycle. Edging techniques can be informed by knowledge of changes in libido, sensitivity, and arousal. Modify edging techniques in accordance with each person's unique hormonal cycle. Some women might find that edging experiences are more possible at particular times of the month.
4. Comfort and Vaginal Lubrication: Recognize the role that vaginal lubrication plays in enhancing sexual pleasure. Sufficient arousal produces natural

lubrication, which enhances comfort and lowers friction when edging.

Recognize that extra lubrication might be helpful for certain women. Trying out different silicone or water-based lubricants can improve comfort and satisfaction in general.

5. Awareness of the Pelvic Floor: Learn about the function of the pelvic floor muscles in facilitating sexual pleasure. Exercises for the pelvic floor, like Kegels, can help with better muscle control. Exercises for the pelvic floor should be included in edging regimens. Increasing the strength of these muscles improves arousal regulation and may help with issues pertaining to tense muscles.

6. Differences in Sensitivity: Recognize that in erogenous zones, women's sensitivity varies. While some people might need more intense stimulation, others might be more sensitive to touch. Adjust edging methods to suit each person's level of sensitivity. Finding the most enjoyable pressure, speed, and pattern can be achieved by experimenting.

7. Aging and Menopause Considerations: Understand that hormonal changes brought on by aging and menopause can impact sexual responses.

Women's edging techniques might need to change to accommodate changing physiological requirements.

Promote candid communication to manage menopause- or aging-related changes, particularly in experiences shared with a partner. This entails having flexibility and modifying strategies as necessary.

C. Developing Self-Confidence:

Developing self-confidence in women who are edging requires a comprehensive strategy that takes into account body image, empowerment, communication, awareness, education, self-care, affirmations that are positive, and community support. Understanding one's desires, accepting oneself as unique, and cultivating an optimistic and self-empowering mindset are the keys to developing confidence.

1.A positive perception of oneself: Encourage body positivity and a positive self-image. Accept and celebrate the individuality of your body, realizing that it deserves respect and affection. Face down societal preconceptions and unattainable beauty standards. Being aware that there are many different types of beauty helps people feel more at ease in their own skin.

2. Sexual Empowerment: Unafraid to accept and own one's desires. Acknowledge that having a sexual desire is a basic and natural aspect of being human.
Encourage yourself to learn about and establish a connection with your own desires. This procedure fosters a feeling of sexual empowerment and boosts self-assurance in general.

3. Skills in Communication: Learn how to communicate effectively so that you can honestly express your needs and boundaries. Building confidence requires open communication with oneself and, if applicable, a partner.
Remain receptive to receiving and providing helpful criticism. A sense of mastery and self-assurance are bolstered by the capacity to modify and improve in response to feedback.

4. Mindfulness Exercises: Remain mindful in order to be in the present. Engaging in edging activities with mindful awareness cultivates a more profound connection with one's body and sensations. Build a solid mental-physical bond. Having a better understanding of how emotions and ideas affect bodily reactions helps one approach edging with greater assurance.

5. Knowledge and Education: Seek thorough sexual education to debunk falsehoods and misconceptions. Women who possess knowledge are better equipped to make educated choices and feel more confident about their sex lives. Recognize the sexual response and anatomy of women. Understanding one's own body gives one more self-assurance when navigating sexual situations, including edging techniques.

6. Consistent Self-Care: Give self-care for both physical and emotional well-being a high priority. Regular exercise, a healthy diet, and stress management help to foster a positive self-image and confidence.
Celebrate personal accomplishments and progress in edging practices. Acknowledging growth and positive experiences helps to reinforce a sense of confidence.

7. Positive Affirmations:Incorporate positive affirmations that affirm self-worth and sexual agency. Remind yourself often that desires are valid and that self-expression is necessary for a fulfilling sexual journey. Actively confront negative thoughts or self-doubt.

8. Community Engagement: Make connections with communities that foster constructive dialogue about sexual orientation. Talking to others about your experiences can help you feel confident and like you belong. Interact with peers who have gone through comparable things. Gaining knowledge from the experiences of others can boost confidence by offering motivation and new perspectives.

D. Exploration of Preferences:

An individualized and flexible strategy is needed to investigate women's edging experiences. Women can overcome obstacles and promote a more fulfilling edging journey by putting an emphasis on personalized exploration, open communication, fantasy integration, variety in stimulation, comfort prioritization, self-reflection, and a commitment to consent and boundaries.

1. Tailored Exploration: Recognize that every woman has different tastes. When it comes to edging, there is no one-size-fits-all method; personal investigation is essential. Try out different edging strategies to see what makes you feel the happiest. Adjust strategies according to individual preferences and reactions.

2. Open Communication: Encourage honest discussion about boundaries, preferences, and desires with your spouse. Starting a conversation guarantees that experiences with partnered edging correspond with personal preferences. Women should be encouraged to speak up for their preferences and needs. Speaking up about what works and what needs to be adjusted makes edging more enjoyable.

3. Fantasy and Mental Engagement: Examine how to incorporate imagination and mental activity when edging. Including private fantasies can raise arousal and help with a more enjoyable experience. Pay attention to how your mental activity affects your level of arousal. Grasping the significance of imagination in individual choices contributes a mental aspect to edging behaviors.

4. Stimulation Variability: Stress how important it is to use a variety of stimulation methods. Individual preferences can be accommodated by adjusting pressure, speed, patterns, and concentrating on distinct erogenous zones. Constantly ask for feedback and make changes according to what makes you feel the happiest. By going through this iterative process, edging

practices are made to conform to changing preferences.

5. Security and Comfort: When edging, put your own comfort and safety first. A more leisurely and pleasurable exploration of preferences is made possible by a sense of security and comfort. Try out new methods little by little. Gradual investigation offers the chance to evaluate preferences without overwhelming sensations.

6. Introspection: Promote introspection following edging encounters. Examine the elements that you found enjoyable, uncomfortable, or that could be changed to accommodate changing preferences. Tastes can change over time. Be willing to modify your edging techniques in response to shifting preferences and comfort zones.

7. Agreement and Limitations: Be sure to express consent and boundaries clearly. Edging experiences respect personal boundaries and preferences when clear guidelines are established. Continue to communicate with your partners about your preferences, making sure they are informed of any changes or special requests. An atmosphere of harmony and consensus is fostered by this continuing conversation.

E. Practice and Patience:

Overcoming obstacles in women's edging experiences requires both persistent practice and patience. Women can successfully navigate challenges and eventually achieve a more satisfying edging journey by being aware of the learning curve, committing to regular practice, maintaining mindful awareness, adapting approaches, managing expectations, reinforcing positive efforts, and seeking support when needed.

1. Acknowledging the Learning Process:.Recognize that edging has a learning curve just like any other skill. Recognize that self-improvement requires time and experience, and exercise patience with yourself. Acknowledge incremental gains and advancements over time. No matter how small the improvement, acknowledging it helps one maintain a positive outlook.

2. Regular Engagement: Adhere to regular practice sessions. The regular application of edging techniques facilitates the growth of comfort, familiarity, and a more profound comprehension of preferences. Include edging in your regular self-care routines. Frequent sessions help the process become more comfortable over time and help to establish a sense of normalcy.

3. Consciousness: While edging, cultivate mindful awareness. A more immersive and pleasurable experience is made possible by being in the present moment, which also strengthens the mind-body connection. Seize the chance to learn from every edging session. During the practice, take note of what goes well, what could be changed, and how the sensations change.

4. Adaptive Methodology: Be prepared to modify methods in response to changing comfort levels and preferences. A personalized experience and ongoing improvement are made possible by a flexible approach.
Be willing to investigate novel edging techniques. Experimenting with various methods can reveal latent preferences and lead to a more satisfying practice.

5. Controlling Anticipations: Establish reasonable goals for your progress. Acknowledge that every person's experience with edging is different and that progress might take some time. Welcome to the journey of discovery and learning. Resilience and patience are fostered when obstacles are seen as chances for personal development.

6. Self-Encouragement: Engage in self-affirmation and constructive criticism. To increase self-confidence and motivation, remind yourself of your accomplishments, no matter how tiny. Express gratitude for the work you've put into learning edging techniques. A positive outlook is reinforced by acknowledging the dedication to personal development.

7. Looking for Assistance and Direction: If challenges continue, think about getting expert advice. Counselors or sex therapists can offer customized approaches and assistance in getting through particular challenges.
Make connections with encouraging groups where people exchange stories and wisdom. Gaining inspiration and useful advice from the experiences of others can be obtained.

Women's edging strategies include customized arousal exploration that integrates experimentation, communication, and mindfulness. Women can improve their experiences, both alone and in relationships, by embracing their unique preferences and overcoming obstacles in order to prolong their enjoyment and contentment.

Communication and Consent in Mutual Edging

Consent, boundaries, open communication, and clear communication are essential components that guarantee couples a positive, consensual, and fulfilling mutual edging experience. In order to negotiate the complexities of desire, preferences, and boundaries with trust and understanding, partners need to create a safe and open communication environment.

A. Establish Clear Communication

1. Planning and Goals: Talk about your intentions prior to starting a mutual edging exchange. Talk about what each partner wants to get out of the session, discover, or accomplish.
Deal with any worries or anxieties.
To facilitate communication, create a relaxed atmosphere where both partners can freely express their opinions.

2. Preferences and Desires: Promote candid communication about preferences. It is important for both partners to communicate what they find

enjoyable, thought-provoking, or exciting in order
to better understand one another's preferences.
Engage in active hearing. Make sure that neither
partner interrupts or passes judgment on the other
while they actively listen to their wants, worries,
and expectations.

3. Feedback Mechanism: Create a system for
providing feedback both during and following the
edging encounter. Invite partners to share their
thoughts after the session as well as their
immediate feedback on what went well and what
could be improved. Encourage productive dialogue.
If changes are required, present recommendations
in an upbeat and encouraging way, emphasizing
your mutual satisfaction and enjoyment.

B. Boundaries and Consent:

1. Setting Boundaries: During the edging session,
clearly define each person's boundaries. Talk about
particular methods, approaches, or domains that
are forbidden or might call for additional consent
and communication. Throughout the session,
periodically check in with each other to make sure
that boundaries are being respected. This
continuous exchange of messages maintains a
mutually satisfying and consensual experience.

2. Consent Dynamics: Stress the value of verbal and nonverbal clues in obtaining consent. Even though spoken communication is important, it's important to observe nonverbal clues that convey comfort or discomfort. Think about putting in place a safe word system. If one partner feels the need to stop or pause, using a safe word ensures that the interaction is courteous and consensual.

3. Permission for Modifications: Recognize that tastes and comfort zones might shift throughout the session. A mutual understanding should be established so that each partner can modify or halt activities in response to changing feelings. Make sure that when boundaries or preferences change, both partners feel comfortable communicating those changes. A sense of agency and control over the edging experience are enhanced by this empowerment.

4. Post-Session Communication: Talk to each other after the session. Discuss what went well, what could be done better, and any new information discovered from the mutual edging experience. Make use of the post-session talks to talk about future session boundaries. Boundaries are consistently respected when there is continuous

communication, even though preferences may change over time.

Creating a Shared Edging Experience
A. Symmetric Participation

Both partners actively participate in and steer the edging experience when there is equal engagement in symmetrical participation. Couples create a shared edging experience that enables intimacy, exploration, and mutual satisfaction through shared responsibility, taking turns, diversity in techniques, feedback and adjustment, mutual empowerment, emotional connection, and mindful presence.

1. Equitable Contribution and Shared Responsibilities: Stress how critical it is that both partners take an active role in the edging process. When both parties participate, a sense of shared responsibility is created and a balanced contribution is guaranteed. Try to prevent any unequal participation by making sure that each partner has an equal chance to lead, explore, and enjoy the session.

2. Switching Roles: Promote the idea that you will alternate between being the "edger" and the person who is feeling the edge. Both partners will have an

equal chance to guide and be guided thanks to this reciprocal approach. Couples can investigate edging dynamics from both viewpoints by switching roles. This fosters empathy and understanding between people, making the experience more shared and compassionate.

3. Variety of Methods: Together, explore with various edging methods. The pace, pressure, and focus should be actively explored with by both partners, according to their individual preferences. View the edging session as a group exploration. A collaborative environment that encourages exploration is created when both partners actively engage in trying new things.

4. Feedbacks and Modifications: Set up a dual feedback mechanism in which each partner shares their thoughts on what works, what needs to be changed, and what they would prefer to do next. This guarantees that providing feedback is a cooperative and shared. Promote responsiveness to each other's feedback.
A dynamic and adaptable shared experience is created when both partners actively listen to each other and modify their approach in response to the cues given.

5. Mutual Empowerment: Throughout the experience, promote equitable control dynamics. To establish a shared sense of control, both partners should feel empowered to direct the edging experience's intensity, pacing, and focus. Empowering one another reciprocally helps to foster a sense of mutual confidence. Each partner actively participates in and values the other's desires fostering a trusting and positive relationship.

6. Emotional Bonding: The emotional bond is strengthened by reciprocal involvement. Couples forge a shared narrative that deepens their relationship by actively exploring each other's desires. Participation that is symmetrical makes the experience feel more personal. The mutual engagement and shared responsibility cultivate a feeling of intimacy and connection that deepens the emotional experience of the shared edging journey.

7. Contemplative Presence: Engage in a cooperative mindful awareness while edging. In order to establish a shared and in-the-moment connection, both partners actively concentrate on the feelings, thoughts, and responses. Discuss your shared experience after the session. Talk about the parts that both of you enjoyed, any new information you

learned, and how the interaction enhanced the intimacy of the experience.

B. Taking Turns:
1. Creating a Reciprocal Dynamic: Stress the idea that each person should alternate between being the "edger" and the person feeling the edge. By creating a reciprocal dynamic, you can be sure that each partner actively participates in leading and enjoying the session.
Role switching keeps control dynamics in balance. A more balanced and cooperative experience is produced by giving each partner the chance to take on the roles of both giver and receiver.

2. Comparative Examination: Both partners can exchange perspectives by taking turns. The receiver investigates the range of ways they can react and express their desires, while the "edger" learns more about the sensations they offer.

This exchange of ideas turns into a cooperative educational process. Couples figure out what suits them best fostering a deeper understanding of preferences and enhancing the overall shared journey.

3. Encouraging Both Partners: By taking turns, both partners are able to actively contribute to leading the session. Sharing control fosters equality and a sense of shared accountability for the edging experience between the giver and the recipient. As each partner actively participates in providing and receiving pleasure, their confidence grows. An environment of positivity and trust is fostered by this shared empowerment between partners.

C. Variety in Techniques:
This includes experimenting with tools and sensation play, incorporating internal techniques, changing tempo and rhythms, exploring different stimulation methods, trying out different edging techniques, encouraging open communication and feedback, integrating fantasy, incorporating role play, and adjusting to each other's reactions. The shared edging experience is made more dynamic, interesting, and suited to the preferences of both partners by this variety.

1. Exploring Various Stimulation Techniques: Clitoral Stimulation: Try out different clitoral stimulation methods. Different sensations can be obtained by varying pressure, speed, and patterns, giving both partners a varied experience.

Exploration of Erogenous Zones: Continue the investigation into additional erogenous zones. Find places that react differently to various forms of touch, adding to the shared edging experience's overall diversity.

2. Internal Stimulation Methods: When a partner feels comfortable exploring this kind of exploration, introduce them to internal stimulation techniques. Try varying the angles, rhythms, and intensities to see what makes you more happy. When integrating internal stimulation, constant communication is essential. During this part of the shared edging experience, partners should be transparent about their preferences, comfort zones, and any necessary adjustments.

3. Changing Rhythms and Pacing: Try varying how quickly the stimulation is provided. A dynamic and captivating experience can be produced for both the giver and the recipient by switching between slower and faster rhythms. When partners are switching roles, synchronize rhythms. A feeling of anticipation and pleasure is shared by both parties, which strengthens the connection.

4. Tools and Sensation Play: Present sensation play by exploring with various materials and temperatures. This can add a layer of novelty to the shared edging experience, such as feather touches, ice, or even warming sensations. Before using any tools or sensation play components, make sure that express consent has been obtained. To establish a relaxed and cooperative environment, talk about boundaries and preferences.

5. Trying Out Different Edging Methods: Consider using the start-stop method, which involves pausing stimulation prior to reaching climax. This enhances the shared edging experience by creating anticipation and prolonging the pleasure. Try the squeeze technique, which entails applying light pressure to the clitoral region or base of the penis. This method can postpone the orgasm and give the shared experience a new depth.

6. Feedback and Communication: Encourage partners to discuss their preferences and reactions to various techniques in an honest and open manner. This dialogue guarantees that changes can be made to accommodate personal preferences.

Following each technique, swap feedback. Talk about the enjoyable aspects, the things that could be changed, and any fresh concepts to investigate. The collaborative aspect of the shared edging experience is strengthened by reciprocal feedback.

7. Incorporating Fantasy: Include shared fantasies in the process of edging. Talk honestly about your fantasies and desires to create an environment where both parties can explore and become more aroused. During the edging session, partners can describe fantasies through verbalization and imagery. This gives the experience a mental component that strengthens the variety and connection.

8. Incorporating Role Play: Try switching roles during the edging procedure. Assign roles to each other so that the dynamics can change and new insights into pleasure can arise. When implementing role play, it is imperative to communicate clearly. It is important for partners to be honest about their comfort zones, personal space, and any particular situations they would like to explore.

9. Adjusting to Each Other's Response: Constantly modify methods according to each other's reactions. Be aware of nonverbal clues as well as spoken ones, and adapt to your partner's shifting comfort zones and desires. Develop a repertoire of enjoyable techniques with your partner over time. A variety of strategies build a toolkit for a fulfilling and varied shared edging experience.

Strengthening Intimacy through Mutual Control

A. Shared Control Dynamics:
Equitable decision-making, switching roles, reciprocal responsiveness, empowering both partners, open communication during control shifts, cultivating an emotional bond, collaborative mindful presence, and reflection with reciprocal aftercare are all examples of shared control dynamics that strengthen intimacy.
A cooperative, mutually agreeable, and deeply emotional shared edging experience is enhanced by these components.

1. Equitable Decision-Making: In shared control dynamics, decisions made during the edging experience are actively participated in by both partners. Assign equal control to each person so

that they can both contribute equally to the direction of the meeting. In order to promote cooperation and shared accountability, decisions should be made with the consent of both parties. An agreed-upon and shared approach to the intimate encounter is facilitated by this balance.

2. Taking Turns Leading: Encourage participants to take turns running the session. To ensure that both parties experience the power and vulnerability inherent in mutual control, each partner alternates between being the giver and the receiver. Switching between roles gives both partners reciprocal power. Giving pleasure gives the giver a sense of agency, and receiving it empowers the recipient to direct their own happiness.

3. Equitable Reactivity: Mutual responsiveness is a requirement of shared control. By actively responding to each other's cues, preferences, and feedback, the two partners establish a dynamic and responsive atmosphere. Adaptability is crucial. In order to strengthen the cooperative aspect of shared control, partners should be willing to make changes in response to each other's changing preferences and comfort zones.

4. Establishing a Sense of Empowerment for Both Partners: Both partners feel more empowered when they share control. Every person actively influences and adds to the experience, creating an environment that is uplifting and empowering. Mutual empowerment based on shared control dynamics fosters trust. The intimacy is strengthened overall because both partners have faith in one another to handle the complexities of pleasure, desires, and boundaries.

5. Interaction During Control Transitions: Good communication is essential when there are changes in power. To ensure a smooth and agreeable transition, partners should be very clear about their intentions, desires, and any changes in control. When taking charge, encourage partners to be honest about what they want. By adding a layer of transparency, this communication makes the experience more personal and communal.

6. Bonding on an emotional level: The emotional bond is strengthened when control is shared. As a result of their shared responsibility for leading and enjoying the journey, both partners become mutually invested in it. Vulnerability is a part of navigating control dynamics. By being vulnerable with one another and putting their trust in one

another's desires and reactions, partners strengthen their relationship.

7. Collaborative Mindful Presence: Joint mindful presence enhances shared control. To strengthen their relationship, both partners actively concentrate on the feelings, thoughts, and actions in the here and now.
Having a mindful presence encourages group exploration. Together, partners actively participate in the experience, forging a shared story that deepens their emotional bond.

8. Aftercare and Reflection: Encourage partners to discuss the shared control dynamics in a group after the session. Talk about the positive aspects of the experience, the difficulties encountered, and how it enhanced the intimacy overall.
Take part in aftercare with one another. Take care of each other's emotional health by offering consolation and encouragement. The caring and shared nature of the intimate encounter is reinforced by this post-session care.

B. Empowerment and Trust:
In mutual control, empowerment and trust entail equitable involvement, cooperative decision-making, confidence-building, navigating

vulnerability with trust, cooperative inquiry, cultivating emotional bonding, actively empowering one another, and giving thoughtful feedback. Together, these components foster a mutually agreeable, empowering, and trust-fostering atmosphere that enhances the intimacy of the shared edging experience.

1. Mutual Empowerment: Equitable participation is the first step toward empowerment in mutual control. To guarantee that one does not control the other in making decisions, both partners actively participate in leading and enjoying themselves. Give each person a feeling of agency. During the edging experience, each partner should have the confidence to voice their wants, take initiative, and actively participate in the dynamics of shared control.

2. Joint Decision-Making: Promote working together to make decisions. To create a shared and consensual edging experience, partners should make decisions together, taking into account each other's preferences, comfort levels, and desires. Make certain that each partner has an equal voice in the decisions made during the meeting. This equality stops one partner from controlling the

decision-making process and encourages mutual empowerment.

3. Developing Self-Belief: Give encouragement and supportive feedback. By recognizing and appreciating each partner's choices, efforts, and active participation, you can boost self-esteem and confidence. Recognize the efforts put forth by each partner to manage shared control. Mutual appreciation for one another's contributions enhances the dynamic of empowerment as a whole.

4. Vulnerability Trust: Having shared control makes one vulnerable. As both partners navigate and expose themselves physically and emotionally, trust is developed. Intimacy is fostered and the connection is strengthened by trust in vulnerability. Communication that is open and honest builds trust. To build a foundation of trust in one another's intentions, partners should be honest in communicating their wants, boundaries, and concerns.

5. Exploration with Consent: Explicit consent strengthens trust and empowerment. It is important for both partners to actively consent to every aspect of the edging experience in order to

establish mutual agreement and ensure that boundaries are respected.

Throughout the session, use ongoing check-ins to confirm consent. Regular communication fosters a respectful and consensual atmosphere, which strengthens trust.

6. Emotional Bond: A shared emotional investment is necessary for mutual control dynamics to occur. The emotional parts of the edging experience are actively invested in and contributed to by both partners, strengthening their bond.

As couples navigate each other's pleasures and desires, trust is built. A bond is formed as a result of the shared responsibility, encouraging confidence in one another's ability to lead and tend to personal needs.

7. Encouraging One Another: Establish a nurturing environment where partners actively support and empower one another. During the shared control dynamics, encourage each other to speak in a way that is affirming and upbeat, thereby boosting their confidence and self-esteem. Throughout the session, actively support one another. Mutual empowerment is fostered by complimenting, expressing gratitude, and recognizing the positive aspects of each other's contributions.

8. Contemplation and Input: Have thoughtful
conversations following the edging session. Talk
about your thoughts, feelings, and the entire
experience. This contemplation strengthens the
sense of empowerment and trust that arises from
the dynamics of shared control. During the
post-session reflection, give encouragement. In
order to continue a positive cycle of empowerment
and trust for upcoming interactions, acknowledge
the positive aspects of shared control.

C. Developing Intimacy:
Developing intimacy through mutual control entails
developing a physical and emotional bond,
establishing shared rituals, fostering a shared
emotional investment, mutual trust and
transparency, collaborative decision-making,
empathetic understanding, mindful presence, and
reciprocal empowerment. During the shared edging
experience, these components help partners
develop a strong and meaningful connection.

1. Shared Emotional Investment: Starting with a
shared emotional investment, mutual control can
be used to build intimacy. In order to lay the
groundwork for a deeper level of connection, both
partners actively engage emotionally. Promote the
disclosure of vulnerabilities. Mutual control

dynamics give couples a safe space to discuss and work through their vulnerabilities, which promotes emotional intimacy.

2. Transparency and Trust: Open communication is the foundation of intimacy. Establish a forum where partners can freely discuss their needs, wants, and boundaries. This openness strengthens the emotional bond and fosters trust. Encourage partners to be open and honest about their expectations and desires. By being honest, you both develop a greater awareness of each other's personal needs, which fortifies your emotional connection.

3. Joint Decision-Making: Intimacy-building calls for collaborative decision-making. Throughout the edging process, both partners actively participate in decision-making, fostering a cooperative environment and a sense of shared accountability. Make sure that choices are mutually agreed upon and represent the preferences of both parties. This cooperative process of reaching decisions strengthens the emotional bond and adds to a common story.

4. Empathic comprehension: Encourage understanding with empathy. In order to foster an environment that supports and fosters emotional intimacy, partners should actively acknowledge and comprehend one another's points of view. Acknowledge and validate each other's feelings. Recognize and value the spectrum of feelings that are encountered during shared control dynamics in order to strengthen a compassionate and understanding relationship.

5. Mindful Presence: Being mindful of the present moment enhances intimacy. To foster a stronger bond by actively participating in the shared moment, encourage partners to be mindful and totally present during the edging experience. Include group mindfulness exercises. Mutual awareness practices, breathing exercises, and guided meditation all help create a synchronized and personal experience.

6. Empowering Each Other: Intimacy is cultivated through reciprocal empowerment. In order to acknowledge and value each other's contributions during the shared control dynamics, partners should actively empower one another. Honor each other's autonomy and uniqueness. Recognize each partner's special abilities and contributions to the

close relationship in order to foster a feeling of intimacy and appreciation.

7. Post-Session Analysis: Have thoughtful conversations following the edging session. By exchanging ideas, feelings, and criticism, partners can better comprehend one another's viewpoints and experiences. Show your appreciation for the shared experience. Recognize and value the emotional openness, trust, and participation that were displayed throughout the session, creating a feeling of positivity and community.

8. Emotional and Physical Ties: Physical intimacy is frequently displayed. As partners actively participate in enjoying and being pleased, the shared control dynamics forge a special physical bond that strengthens the physical bond. Emotional attachment is facilitated by mutual control's physical actions. Intimacy is increased overall because of the shared vulnerability and responsibility, which forge an emotional connection beyond physical feelings.

9. Establishing Common Practices and Rituals: Create customs that you both follow during the edging process. Establishing shared practices, whether they be verbal affirmations, particular

techniques, or unconventional approaches, promotes a feeling of closeness and familiarity. These shared rituals' consistency strengthens the emotional bond. Maintaining intimacy is facilitated by shared practices and a sense of security that comes with knowing what to expect.

D. Mindful Presence in Developing Mutual Control and Intimacy:

1. Present-Moment Focus: Being mindfully present means focusing on the here and now. During the edging experience, encourage both partners to actively use their senses, completely experiencing the feelings, connections, and sensations in the present. Include breathing in synchrony. By synchronizing their breathing, couples can establish a shared rhythm that improves mindfulness and strengthens their bond.

2. Intense Perception: The sensory experience is enhanced by mindful presence. To create a more immersive and intimate encounter, encourage partners to focus on the touch, scent, taste, and sounds that are involved in the shared control dynamics. With a spirit of appreciation and curiosity, actively examine each other's bodies. There is an increased awareness of the physical and

emotional connection when there is mindful touch and exploration.

3. Observation Without Judgment: Develop an impartial sense of observation. Partners should create an environment of acceptance and understanding by observing each other's reactions, desires, and expressions without passing judgment. Make sure the surroundings support impartial observation. Partners should be able to express themselves without worrying about being judged, fostering a thoughtful and caring environment.

4. Sensitivity to Emotions: Recognizing emotional reactions is part of being mindfully present. Being aware of one's own and the other's feelings will help both partners build a stronger emotional bond during the shared control dynamics. Inspire your partners to express their feelings through words. Real-time sharing of emotional experiences fosters more connected and open communication, which improves the encounter's general mindfulness.

5. Collaborative Mindfulness Exercises: Practice breathing exercises together. By coordinating their breathing, couples can engage in a cooperative mindfulness exercise that strengthens their bond and encourages a shared experience. Throughout

the session, introduce guided mindfulness moments. These can involve brief stops for cooperative concentration, establishing deliberate instances of shared awareness throughout the encounter.

6. Establishing an Environment Free from Distractions: Distraction-free environments foster mindful presence. In order to create a space where they can fully focus on each other and the shared control dynamics, encourage partners to reduce external distractions.
Take into consideration shutting down or muting electronic gadgets. This small gesture creates a more contemplative atmosphere that enables partners to fully enjoy the intimate moment.

7. Expressions of Thanks and Appreciation: Expressing gratitude for the shared experience is a part of mindful presence. It is possible for both partners to express gratitude for one another's presence, contributions, and the bond that was created during the mutual control dynamics.

Encourage partners to consider the positive aspects of their experience during the post-session reflection. By concentrating on intimate and enjoyable moments, the interaction becomes more mindful and appreciative.

8. Conscientious Shifts: The practice of mindful presence includes changing roles. Partners should carefully manage these changes, whether they are going from giver to receiver or the other way around, to guarantee a seamless and mutually agreeable change in power.

For couples, mutual edging entails good communication, building a shared experience, and enhancing intimacy via shared control. Couples can improve their emotional bond and design a deeper and more fulfilling edging journey together by embracing mutual control dynamics, communicating clearly and giving consent, and actively participating in the shared experience.

Chapter Five: Overcoming Challenges in Edging

Typical Obstacles with Edging

A. Insufficient Patience when Edging:
An important obstacle in the edging process is impatience, which makes it hard for people to wait for satisfaction and tempts them to go for an orgasm too soon.

Approach:
Using Mindfulness Practices to Develop Patience: This method helps create a more thoughtful and connected intimate relationship in addition to addressing the immediate problem of impatience.

1. Mindful Breathing:Mindful breathing entails paying attention to the breath and taking slow, deliberate breaths in and out. It encourages people to breathe deeply and mindfully while they are edging. This exercise helps people become more at ease and diverts their focus from their impatience.

2. Present-Moment Awareness: Living in the present without getting sucked into fantasies or expectations about the future. It helps people direct their attention to the feelings and experiences that

are occurring right now. This can be accomplished
by encouraging them to express their feelings and
experiences verbally.

3. Sensory Engagement: This involves using the
senses in a deliberate manner to increase awareness
of the body's experiences. It encourages your
partner to experiment with various temperatures,
textures, and forms of touch. This sensory
interaction helps to divert attention from
impatience while also enhancing experience variety.

4. Mindful Arousal Observation: This is keeping an
objective eye on arousal levels while avoiding haste
or judgment. It helps people notice how their
arousal levels rise and fall. This exercise cultivates a
nonjudgmental mindset toward the process and
makes them more conscious of their own reactions.

5. Guided Imagery: This involves concentrating
attention and reducing impatience by visualizing or
imagining a situation. This encourages partners to
visualize a situation that will increase their level of
pleasure during guided imagery.
This mental activity can help create a more
immersive experience and serve as a diversion from
impatience.

6. Progressive Muscle Relaxation: This encourages general relaxation, systematically tense and relax various muscle groups. While edging, incorporate progressive muscle relaxation exercises. This method lessens tension both physically and mentally, calming the mind and fostering patience.

7. Communication Breaks: This one is about taking short breaks to discuss and evaluate feelings. Throughout the edging experience, encourage partners to take brief breaks to share their experiences with one another. Expressing emotions through words can aid impatience management and encourage teamwork.

8. Realistic Expectations Setting: About specifying realistic expectations and goals for the edging session.
This assist individuals and groups in establishing reasonable expectations. Managing impatience is made easier by realizing that edging is a gradual process that may require trial and error.

9. Establishing a Mindful Routine: For edging sessions, establish a regular, mindful routine. Developing a routine aids in people's familiarization and comfort level with the

procedure. Impatience can be lessened by repetition by fostering a sense of predictability.

10. Gratitude Practice: During the edging process, concentrate on the good things and express gratitude.
Start a gratitude exercise wherein partners express their gratitude for the experience they had together. This encouraging feedback can help people adopt a more appreciative mindset and divert their attention from their impatience.

People can gradually develop patience by using these mindfulness techniques, which will make the edging process more pleasurable and fulfilling.

B. Having Trouble Staying Focused While Edging:

Distractions and daydreaming can interfere with the edging experience and make it difficult for people to keep the required focus.

Approach:
Engage in Mindfulness Activities and Establish a Friendly Environment

1. Deep Breathing: Deep breathing encourages concentration and relaxation by involving slow, deliberate breaths. Start the edging session with deep breathing exercises and continue it throughout. This promotes mindfulness, mental calmness, and attentional refocusing on the here and now.

2. Guided Meditation: Guided meditation helps focus and calm the mind by offering an organized, narrated experience. Introduce guided meditation sessions designed with the experience of edging in mind. This can take the form of spoken instructions or a pre-recorded session that helps people stay focused and in the moment.

3. Mindful Body Scan: To promote awareness and relaxation, one can mentally focus on various body parts by performing a body scan. Focus on every area of your body. This strengthens the connection to physical sensations and helps sustain focus.

4. Visual Anchors: Focusing attention in a different direction by using visual cues or objects as anchors. Add something visually soothing to the surroundings.

To help you focus and reduce distractions, vision anchors should be used as the center of attention during the edging session.

5. Breathing Rhythms: For a soothing and rhythmic effect, match breathing rhythms to particular counts. Incorporate breathing patterns that correspond with the edging experience's speed. This coordinated strategy controls arousal levels in addition to helping with focus.

6. Mindful Touch Exploration: Using your hands to explore while paying attention to feel. Encourage couples to mindfully examine each other's bodies. People can refocus their attention from distracting thoughts to the physical experience by focusing on the tactile sensations.

7. Decluttering the Mind: Recognizing and consciously refocusing attention on distracting thoughts.
Helps people identify distracting thoughts without passing judgment. You should intentionally let go of these interruptions and return your attention to the feelings and experience you are both sharing right now.

8. Mindful Communication Breaks: Taking brief pauses to express emotions and regain focus. Include deliberate pauses in the edging process so that partners can reconnect and talk. Realigning focus and strengthening the bond can both be achieved through verbalizing feelings and experiences.

9. Conducive Environment: Making a space free of pointless interruptions. Encourage creating the edging area in a calm, cozy, and clutter-free setting. Reducing the amount of outside stimuli helps create an environment that encourages prolonged focus.

10. Visualization Methods: Constructing mental pictures or scenarios to direct focus. Introduce partners to visualization exercises where they imagine enjoyable situations in their minds. By using this method, one can improve mental engagement with the experience and divert attention from outside distractions.

In addition to improving focus, these techniques also make intimate experiences more fulfilling and immersive.

C. Barriers in Edging Caused by Emotions:

The enjoyment of the edging process can be hampered by emotional factors that create emotional barriers that impair the entire experience, such as anxiety, stress, or performance pressure.

Approach:

Promote Honesty and Offer Sympathetic Assistance: Setting reasonable goals, using relaxation techniques, exploring, reassurance, open communication, emotional check-ins, mindfulness exercises, loving touch, and post-session reflection are all important aspects of the therapeutic process.

1. Open Communication: Provide a secure and welcoming environment where partners can freely talk about their feelings. People should feel free to voice their opinions and worries regarding the edging procedure. Communicate often in order to comprehend one another's emotional states and deal with any potential worries or anxieties.

2. Emotional Check-Ins: Periodic evaluations of emotional health throughout the edging experience. Provide emotional check-in breaks into your schedule. A supportive environment can be created when partners briefly express their feelings and

make sure that any new feelings are recognized and dealt with.

3. Emotional Exploration: Exploration and understanding one another's emotional reactions. Helps partners investigate the feelings associated with the act of edging. Forging a closer bond can entail talking about fantasies, desires, or any potential emotional triggers.

4. Giving Reassurance: Reducing stress or anxiety by giving both verbal and physical reassurance. Encourage your partners to reassure each other by giving consoling touches or words of affirmation. The emotional experience can be improved and performance pressure can be reduced when individuals are aware of their emotional support system.

5. Mindfulness Practices: Staying present and lowering anxiety through the use of mindfulness techniques. Incorporate mindfulness exercises to assist partners in remaining rooted in the here and now, such as guided meditation or deep breathing. Being mindful can ease tension and foster serenity.

6. Affectionate Touch:Expressing emotional support through a soft and loving touch. Include gentle touch moments to imply connection and emotional support. In order to reduce anxiety and strengthen the emotional connection, physical affection can be a very effective tool.

7. Non-Judgmental Atmosphere: Establishing a setting devoid of criticism and judgment. Stresses the value of providing a safe environment for inquiry. Couples should have a sense of acceptance and encouragement, which will let them express themselves without worrying about backlash.

8. Relaxation Techniques: Reducing emotional tension through the use of relaxation techniques. To aid in partners' relaxation and emotional release, introduce relaxation techniques like progressive muscle relaxation or gentle massage. This may make the process of edging more pleasurable.

9. In order to reduce performance pressure, it is important to set realistic expectations. Set reasonable goals for the edging session in collaboration with your partners. Assuage performance-related stress by highlighting that the main objectives are pleasure and exploration rather than achieving a particular result.

10. Post-Session Emotional Reflection: Reviewing feelings and encounters following the edging experience. After finishing the edging session, encourage partners to talk about their feelings and experiences. By reflecting after the session, you can strengthen your emotional bond and take advantage of the chance to talk about any unanswered issues.

People can develop a more encouraging and emotionally fulfilling edging experience by using these techniques to negotiate and get through emotional obstacles.

D. Inconsistent Edging Techniques:

Applying edging techniques inconsistently can impede progress and cause frustration. The efficacy of the edging experience may be impacted by the absence of a standardized method.

Approach:

Establish a Regular Schedule and Try Out Different Approaches: A more consistent and satisfying edging experience can be achieved by creating an organized routine, trying out different strategies, keeping lines of communication open about preferences, giving feedback, recording successful techniques, setting goals, choosing joint techniques, managing time well, adapting techniques, and encouraging flexibility.

1. Creating a Routine: Plan out an organized and regular schedule for the edging sessions. Together with your partner, decide on a precise order of action for each edging session. Warm-up exercises, exploration, and a gradual build-up can all be a part of this regimen, which offers a defined structure for consistency.

2. Exploration Sessions: Set aside times to experiment with various edging methods. Set aside particular times to practice different edging methods. This enables couples to experiment with various strategies and determine which ones are most effective for them both and ensuring a more personalized experience.

3. Sharing Preferences: Talk about and share your likes, dislikes, and preferences on a regular basis. Promote candid discussion about the methods and strategies that each partner finds enjoyable. Frequent check-ins regarding preferences help to foster mutual understanding and guarantee that expectations are in line for both parties.

4. Feedback Sessions: Appointed periods for offering input on how well techniques work. Include partner feedback sessions where they can candidly talk about what went well and what needs improvement. This continuous conversation improves the overall experience and helps to improve the edging strategy.

5. Recording Effective Techniques: Make a note of the techniques that lead to satisfying experiences. Motivate partners to record effective pleasurable-enhancing techniques. This can be a straightforward journal or a shared document that serves as a resource for future references for future sessions and maintaining consistent approach.

6. Goal Setting: Establish goals for every edging session in concert with others. Together with your partner, decide on clear objectives for each session, such as extending arousal, discovering novel sensations, or reaching a certain control level. A more concentrated and reliable edging experience is enhanced by well-defined objectives.

7. Cooperative Method Selection: Consensus on the methods to be used in a session. Discuss and decide together which techniques to use before each session. By ensuring that both parties are at ease

with the selected course of action, this promotes a cooperative and consistent experience.

8. Scheduling:Set aside specific time for every stage of the edging procedure. Make sure there is enough time allotted for every stage of the edging procedure. This covers the pre-warm-up, investigation, and the build up phase. Effective time management contributes to a consistent and well paced experience.

9. Adapting Techniques: Be flexible in how you apply techniques in response to different responses from people. Recognize that responses and preferences could change over time. To keep the edging experience personalized and consistent, be willing to modify tactics in response to feedback and personal comfort.

10. Flexibility in Approach: Give the general strategy some leeway.
Even though consistency is essential, give yourself some leeway. Acknowledge that every session might be different from the next, and being flexible guarantees that the edging experience stays lively and sensitive to each person's needs.

Individuals and couples can overcome the difficulty of inconsistent edging techniques by putting these strategies into practice.

E. Lack of Communication in Edging:
Misunderstandings during edging may result from inefficient communication about preferences, limits, or comfort zones, which may negatively affect the experience and satisfaction in general.

Approach:
Encourage Direct and Sincere Communication
A more transparent, cooperative, and fulfilling edging experience can be achieved by establishing a communication framework, carrying out pre-session check-ins, expressing desires, defining boundaries, identifying non-verbal cues, implementing consent checkpoints, holding regular emotional check-ins, holding feedback sessions, mutual goal-setting, and having reflective conversations.

1. Creating a Communication Framework. Prior to and during edging sessions, lay the groundwork for open communication. Partners should be encouraged to create a framework for talking about comfort zones, boundaries, and desires. Developing

a safe word or signal to express discomfort or the need for adjustment is one way to do this.

2. Pre-Session Check-Ins: Have quick conversations to set expectations prior to each edging session. Before starting an edging session, partners should have a brief check-in to talk about any particular needs, worries, or preferences. By doing this, it is ensured that everyone is prepared for the experience and is on the same page.

3. Vocalizing Want: Encourage partners to be honest about what they want. Encourage the creation of an atmosphere in which people are at ease expressing their wants. This may consist of discussing fantasies, specific techniques or activities that enhance pleasure.

4. Establishing Clearly Defined Boundaries: Clearly state and convey your own boundaries. Make sure you both know exactly what your boundaries are. This could entail talking about methods or activities that are forbidden or uncomfortable. For edging to be enjoyable, these boundaries must be respected.

5. Non-Verbal Cues: Throughout the session, be aware of and interpret non-verbal cues. It is important for partners to observe one another's

nonverbal cues, such as their body language and facial expressions. Having a keen sense of these cues allows one to adapt in the moment, which enhances communication.

6. Consent Checkpoints: Schedule planned breaks for discussion and explicit consent. Throughout the edging session, introduce deliberate breaks where partners can expressly check in on each other's comfort and consent levels. This guarantees the security of both parties and control throughout the experience.

7. Regular Emotional Check-Ins: Talking about emotional health both before and after edging. Plan quick emotional check-ins to talk about each partner's feelings as the edging process progresses. In addition to fostering an emotional bond, this facilitates early resolution of any new issues.

8. Feedback Sessions: Set aside time to offer comments on the way the communication is going. Participate in feedback sessions with a communication-specific focus after every session. Determine what went well in terms of expressing boundaries and desires, and what needs to be improved.

9. Mutual Goal Setting: Establish cooperative objectives to ensure efficient correspondence. Determine collaboratively what the communication objectives are for every meeting. This could entail enhancing the overall dynamic of communication, becoming more perceptive of non-verbal clues, or making spoken expressions more clear.

10. Reflective Conversations: Talk about and consider your experiences with communication after edging. After edging sessions, encourage partners to have thoughtful discussions. This offers a chance to discuss any unspoken ideas, exchange insights, and continuously improve communication in preparation for upcoming meetings.

Through the application of these communication tactics, people can surmount the obstacle of inadequate communication in edging.

Techniques to Overcoming Premature Ejaculation or Difficulties in Reaching Orgasm

1. Start-Stop Technique:.Incorporate the start-stop method, which involves pausing stimulation prior to reaching a peak. By using this technique, you can develop control and postpone orgasm.

2. Squeeze Technique: Try the squeeze method, which entails applying light pressure to the clitoral region or the base of the penis. This can lengthen the edging experience and momentarily suppress arousal.

3. Exercises for the Pelvic Floor: Include exercises for the pelvic floor to improve your control over your pelvic muscles. Enhancing the strength of these muscles can help improve control and postpone ejaculation.

4. Pay Attention to Different Sensations:.Temporarily divert attention from genital stimulation. Investigate additional erogenous zones and engage in non-genital contact to increase arousal and reduce pressure.

5. Patterns of Masturbation: Try out various patterns of masturbation. By experimenting with different methods, pressures, and speeds, people can learn more about their own arousal thresholds and possibly get past obstacles to orgasm.

6. Psychological Methodologies: Explore psychological strategies like fantasy integration and visualization. Enhancing arousal and addressing

mental barriers can be achieved through mindful engagement with fantasies or positive imagery.

7. Breath Management: Incorporate breathing exercises. In order to overcome difficulties associated with premature ejaculation, slow, deep breaths can help control arousal levels and encourage relaxation.

8. Incorporate Fantasy: To raise arousal, bring up shared fantasies. Mutually exploring one's fantasies and desires can clear the mind and make it easier to experience an orgasm.

9. Relaxation and Patience: Stress relaxation and patience. Anxiety or the need to orgasm can be detrimental. Promote a carefree attitude and the knowledge that enjoyment and discovery are the main objectives.

10. Mutual Exploration: Take part in mutual criticism. Together, couples can try out various methods and pastimes to find what makes them feel good and helps them get over obstacles.

Addressing typical roadblocks like impatience, staying focused, emotional barriers, inconsistent technique, and lack of communication is necessary to overcome edging challenges.

Certain techniques like start-stop and squeeze, pelvic floor exercises, focus on other sensations, varied masturbation patterns, psychological approaches, breath control, fantasy integration, and emphasizing patience and relaxation are some strategies for dealing with premature ejaculation or difficulties reaching an orgasm.

A successful strategy for overcoming edging challenges involves fostering open communication between partners and customizing these strategies to each partner's preferences.

Exploring Sophisticated Methods for Enhanced Enjoyment

1. Sensory Play: To maximize enjoyment, incorporate sensory elements like temperature play, blindfolding, or the use of textured materials. Examine the ways that sensory stimulation can improve the experience of edging. To increase enjoyment, try varying textures, temperatures, or sensory deprivation methods.

2. Temperature Variations:.To enhance stimulation, use warm or cool sensations when edging. Use things like ice cubes, heated massage oils, or toys that react to temperature changes to incorporate temperature variations. This gives the edging session an extra layer of sensory stimulation.

3. Advanced Erotic Massage Techniques: Develop your arousal by learning and using sophisticated erotic massage techniques.
Explore various erogenous zone-focused massage techniques that can heighten arousal and prolong the edging experience. Include different pressures, strokes and techniques to discover what resonates.

4. Role-play and Fantasy Exploration: To get the mind going, play role-playing games or explore fantasies. During edging, talk about and act out dreams or scenarios. The pleasure is prolonged and arousal is increased by the mental engagement. To ensure a pleasant and consensual experience, make sure there is open communication.

5. Edging with Erotic Media:.To increase arousal, include erotic books, films, or audio files. Try incorporating sensual media into the edging session. Choose reading material that appeals to the interests and fantasies of both parties, as this will increase arousal.

6. Stimulation of the Prostate or G-Spot: Learn sophisticated methods for stimulating the prostate in men or the G-spot in women. Try internal stimulation with your fingers, toys, or specialized devices if it's comfortable for you. This may result in extreme enjoyment and extended edging experience.

7. Tantric Techniques: Gain extended pleasure and increased connection by studying and utilizing tantric practices.
To prolong the edging and strengthen the close relationship, try tantric practices like mindful

touch, prolonged foreplay, and controlled breathing.

8. Edging Challenges: To increase excitement, introduce challenges like fixed positions or restrictions. Provide obstacles for the edging session, such as holding a specific posture or using constraints. These difficulties have the power to heighten the senses and prolong arousal.

Including Penetration into Various Sexual Activities

1. Mutual Masturbation Edging: Participate in mutual masturbation to engage in simultaneous edging. Try edging together while masturbating to each other. This encourages a shared experience and lets partners see how the other reacts to different approaches.

2. Edging During Oral Sex: For an enhanced experience, incorporate edging techniques into oral sex.
During oral sex, incorporate edging techniques by switching between pauses and arousal. This enhances the oral experience with yet another level of pleasure.

3. Edging in Different Positions: Tailor your edging experience by trying out different sexual positions. When edging, experiment with different positions that provide more control and a variety of stimuli. Pleasure can be enhanced by positions that facilitate easy access to erogenous zones.

4. Edging in BDSM Play: For those who are curious about power dynamics, combine edging with BDSM components. Include edging techniques in BDSM plays by introducing concepts such as discipline, dominance, bondage, and submission. Make sure there is consent and clear communication within the BDSM dynamics.

5. Including Toys and Accessory Items: Include sex toys and accessory items to improve edging experiences. Play around with different edging toys, like vibrators, anal plugs, or restraint tools. These extras can lengthen the experience and increase enjoyment.

6. Edging in Outdoor Settings: Examine your experiences edging in various settings, including outdoor ones.
In outdoor settings, experiment with edging if comfort and privacy permit. The experience may

become more exciting and novel due to the change in surroundings.

7. Including Edging in Erotic Games: Include edging in challenges or games involving sex. Create or investigate sensual games with edging obstacles. This may be a fun method to increase anticipation and sustain arousal.

8. Extended Edging Sessions: Commit to edging for the duration of the sessions to ensure sustained enjoyment. Allocate a specific time slot for prolonged edging sessions. This offers the chance to experiment with various methods and experience increased levels of pleasure.

People and partners can improve the overall intimate experience by experimenting with advanced techniques for increased pleasure and edging into various sexual activities. These activities foster inquiry, dialogue, and a closer bond between partners, all of which enhance the satisfaction and fulfillment of a sexual relationship.

Protective Measures and Safety in Edging

The Value of Safe Procedures When Edging:

1. Physical Well-Being: Give emphasis to the physical security and welfare of both edging participants.
Stress the value of staying comfortable and steering clear of potentially harmful activities. An enjoyable and secure edging experience is facilitated by physical well-being consciousness.

2. Communication for Safety: Clearly communicate any safety-related issues. During the edging session, encourage partners to talk honestly about any concerns they may have about safety. This guarantees that changes to address possible risks can be made quickly.

3. Hygiene Practices: Stress the importance of hygiene in order to ward off illnesses or discomfort. Before and during edging, talk about and rank the importance of hygiene practices. This promotes a safe and healthy environment by requiring that hands, the body, and any tools or accessories used during the session be cleaned.

4. Acknowledging Personal Physical Boundaries: Recognize your own personal boundaries to prevent strain or harm. Physical boundaries should be acknowledged and communicated by partners. To avoid pain or injury, don't push your body past its comfortable limits.

5. Safe Word Implementation: If necessary, immediately stop using the safe word or signal. Include a safe word or signal that is well-known and understood by all. This offers a quick and effective way to stop activities if one partner feels unsafe or uneasy.

6. Emotional Safety:.Give your emotional security and wellbeing top priority when edging. Talk about emotional boundaries and make sure that during the edging process, both partners experience emotional security. An experience is more positive and fulfilling when there is emotional safety.

Understanding When to Avoid or Adjust Edging Methods:

1. Pain or Discomfort: Recognize when engaging in certain activities results in pain or discomfort. It's critical to identify any pain or discomfort felt by either partner and adjust the activity appropriately.

Pain may be a sign to steer clear of or modify a particular technique.

2. Physical Limitations: Keep in mind any health issues or physical restrictions. It may be necessary to modify or avoid certain edging techniques if one partner has physical limitations or health concerns. Put your health and safety before particular activities.

3. Medical Considerations: Take into account any specific medical issues that might affect edging. Any pertinent medical conditions or concerns should be discussed between partners. To maintain safety and reduce risks, this information can direct the modification or avoidance of particular edging techniques.

4. Triggers Emotional: Identify and deal with emotional triggers. If engaging in certain activities causes emotional distress, it's critical to discuss and adjust the strategy. Establishing a nurturing atmosphere facilitates couples in managing and steering clear of possible emotional hot spots.

5. Sensitivities or Allergies: Recognize any material or product allergies or sensitivity issues. When choosing equipment, add-ons, or materials for

edging, take any allergies or sensitivities into account. Adjust decisions according to personal sensitivities to ensure safety.

6. Fatigue or Exhaustion: Recognize how fatigue affects edging safety. It is important to consider the possible impact on safety if one partner is worn out or exhausted. To ensure wellbeing, think about reducing the duration or intensity of edging activities.

7. Frequent Health Check-ins: Evaluate general well-being by conducting frequent health check-ins. Talking to each other frequently about their mental and physical health is important. Frequent health check-ins provide an opportunity to talk about any changes that might call for edging procedure adjustments.

8. Educate and Seek Professional Advice: Become knowledgeable about safe practices and, if necessary, seek professional advice. Constantly teach the two partners safe edging techniques. To guarantee a knowledgeable and secure approach, consult professionals, such as therapists or experts in sexual health, if you are unsure or facing difficulties.

Through prioritizing safe practices, fostering transparent communication, and understanding when to alter or forego particular techniques, individuals can establish a setting that places equal emphasis on the physical and emotional well-being of others when edging. For everyone involved, this method helps to ensure a pleasant, cooperative, and secure edging experience.

The Mind-Body Link in Edging

Stressing Mindfulness's Role in Edging

1. Mindfulness Breathing Techniques: Use deliberate, rhythmic breathing to maintain awareness while edging.
Stress the value of mindful breathing in order to improve your awareness of your sensations. Tell people to pay attention to their breathing and time it to the speed at which they are edging.

2. Present-Moment Awareness:.When edging, encourage yourself to remain completely present in the here and now. Encourage people to focus on the sensory experience and keep themselves from being distracted. This entails concentrating on the partner's connection, feelings, and bodily experiences.

3. Sensate Focus:.Pay special attention to specific sensory perceptions and details. Incorporate sensory focus exercises into your edging routine, where participants pay attention to specific sensations like touch, pressure, or temperature. This improves enjoyment and fortifies the link between the mind and body.

4. Include Body Scan Meditation: Include body scan meditation to raise your awareness of your body's sensations. Guide yourself through a body scan, wherein each body part is systematically examined. This increases awareness of one's own body's reactions and fortifies the mind-body link.

5. Visualization Techniques: Use guided imagery or visualization to strengthen the mental connection. Incorporate guided imagery that aligns with the individual's aspirations or dreams. It is possible to raise arousal and the relationship can create a stronger link between mental and physical sensations.

6. Breath Control as a Focus Point; To keep your mind focused, use controlled breathing as a focal point. Learn and know how to anchor the mind and

relax at the same time by using breath control. This aids in maintaining focus on the enjoyable parts of edging.

7. Intentional and Mindful Touch and Exploration: Intentionally and fully engage in touch. Encouraging partners to explore each other's bodies with intention and awareness while edging. This strengthens the relationship between pleasure, touch, and mental presence.

8. Applying Mindfulness Techniques Away From Edging Sessions: Promote mindfulness as a regular habit to improve presence in general. Suggest integrating mindfulness exercises into regular schedules. This can involve practices like yoga, meditation, or simply being present in everyday tasks Regular mindfulness practice contributes to a more meaningful approach to edging.

Linking Sexual Satisfaction and Mental Health

1. Check-ins for Emotional Well-Being: Evaluate emotional well-being on a regular basis both prior to and following edging sessions. Individuals need to consider their emotional states while addressing any worries or anxieties. A comprehensive

approach to edging is encouraged by the link
between sexual satisfaction and emotional
well-being.

2. Positive Affirmations: Increase your sense of
satisfaction and self-worth by using positive
affirmations. Include affirmations that are
empowering regarding one's sexuality and
self-worth. Positive self-talk helps cultivate an
optimistic outlook, which improves the mental
climate for sexual encounters.

3. Resolving Psychological Barriers: Examine and
resolve any psychological obstacles that might
affect your ability to have a satisfying sexual
experience. Establish a secure environment where
you can talk about and overcome psychological
obstacles. This can entail contacting a mental
health expert for support.

4. Stress-Reduction and Pleasure: Stress-reduction
has an effect on sexual satisfaction. You should
learn about how stress management and improved
sex pleasure are related. More fulfilling sex can be
achieved through practices like stress management,
mindfulness, and relaxation.

5. Meditation Exercises:Promote meditation exercises to improve self-awareness. Include contemplative exercises that let you examine your preferences, aspirations, and any elements affecting your mental health. A more fulfilling sexual journey can result from this self-awareness.

6. Holistic Approach to Sexual Health:.Stress the important role that mental health plays in the overall Encourage a sexual health strategy that takes a holistic approach to mental, emotional, and physical health. Understand the importance of mental health as a component of sexual satisfaction.

7. Promoting Open and Mindful Communication with Partner: Encourage partner to communicate in an open and mindful manner. Individuals should be honest with their partners about their needs, wants, and emotional boundaries. In a sexual relationship, understanding and satisfaction are increased when communication is done with mindfulness.

8. Ongoing Education and Research: Encourage an attitude of ongoing education and research regarding sexuality. You should see your sexual journey as an ongoing process of discovery. This

way of thinking lessens the pressure to perform well and promotes a positive relationship between mental health and sexual fulfillment.

Individuals can develop a more profound and satisfying experience by highlighting the part that mindfulness plays in influencing and tying mental health and sexual fulfillment together. This method promotes a comprehensive comprehension of the mind-body connection in the context of sexual pleasure contributing to overall well-being.

Conclusion:

In the exploration of edging, we've delved into key principles that form the foundation of this intimate practice. From understanding the physiological and psychological aspects of arousal to mastering specific edging techniques, the journey has been one of discovery and connection. The importance of mindfulness, communication, and safety has underscored every step, emphasizing a holistic approach to sexual well-being.

We've discussed the significance of edging not merely as a means to delay orgasm but as a pathway to heightened pleasure, deeper connections, and a more profound understanding of one's desires. The intricate interplay between the mind and body has been a recurring theme, highlighting the power of mindfulness in elevating the entire experience.

As we conclude this manual on edging techniques, it's paramount to encourage you, the reader, to embark on your unique journey of exploration. Edging is a personal odyssey, and the techniques outlined are not rigid rules but rather a canvas for you to paint your desires upon. Experimentation is the key to unlocking new realms of pleasure, and discovering your preferences is a continual process.

Embrace the freedom to communicate openly with your partner, fostering an environment where desires, boundaries, and fantasies are shared without judgment. Your sexual journey is dynamic and ever-evolving, and each experience contributes to the tapestry of your intimate connections.

In the realm of edging, there are no strict guidelines—only possibilities waiting to be explored. Find joy in the nuances, relish the sensations, and celebrate the uniqueness of your own desires. Whether you're a novice or a seasoned explorer, the world of edging is vast, and the potential for discovery is boundless.

May this guide serve as a compass, guiding you through the intricacies of edging and empowering you to shape your own narrative of pleasure. Embrace the journey, savor the moments, and let the principles of edging be a catalyst for a richer, more satisfying connection with yourself and your partner.

Happy exploring, and may your intimate journey be filled with pleasure, connection, and a deep understanding of your own desires.